# FAST FOOD
# JUNKY

## PART ONE

*By*

# TRE GARCIA

FAST FOOD JUNKY - Part 1
Copyright © 2018 by Tre Garcia

FIRST EDITION
ISBN-13: 978-0-9980400-0-4 (Print Version)
ISBN-13: 978-0-9980400-1-1 (eBook Version)

www.thefastfoodjunky.com
www.twitter.com/fastfood_Junky
www.instagram.com/fastfood_junky
www.facebook.com/fastfoodjunky

# FAST FOOD
# JUNKY

PART ONE

# CONTENTS

### 3.   THE MIND OF A JUNKY

### 4.   DEATH OF A JUNKY

To my nieces and nephew, thank you for giving me a purpose.
To my sister, thank you for always fighting for me.
To my brother, thank you for forgiving me.
To my mom, thank you for always staying up late, and
helping me write my stories from my Junior High days.
To my dad, thank you for being Superman.

# JUST ANOTHER ORDER

"*Yes! I'll have a super-sized double cheeseburger combo with no onions, and could you add chili cheese to the fries? With a coke.*" I asked the drive-thru attendant.

Staring at the illuminating menu at my local burger joint, I quickly perused through each item like I was some kind of A.I. creation scanning for inventory.

"*Anything else?*" the drive-thru attendant asked.

"*Yes,* **WE'LL** *also take a number 11 breakfast sandwich, and also a fudge supreme cake,*" I stated.

This was the part of the drive-thru order when I substituted the contraction of "I'll for **WE'LL**," so that I could give the perception to the drive-thru attendant that all this food couldn't possibly be for one person. Silly? Maybe, but honestly, it was necessary, so I could feel better about inhaling this fast food feast without beating myself to sleep even more than I already did every night.

"*Will that be all?*" The drive-thru attendant asked.

"*...um... yes.*" I said.

I must admit that I could've added an extra breakfast sandwich, but the idea of walking into my parents' home with three greasy bags was shameful enough— imagine a fourth.

# JUST ANOTHER MANIC MONDAY

*L*IFE AS A 401-POUND beast isn't so much for the weak, but mostly for those who simply have no answers. That may sound strange because everywhere I look I'm bombarded with ads of every diet system under the moon, while also being bombarded with advertisements of every fast food joint under the sun. I'm not condoning this as a valid excuse. Believe me when I say this: Every plus size human being on Earth knows when they've reached a new threshold in their size; whether it be: another notch on their belt, change of attire, or the most common characteristic— sporting the same three solid black t-shirts every week for many years to come. Considering all those examples of physical expansion, it's always compounded by telling myself: "This Monday, I'll start eating better and get back into my old clothing in no time."

For me, I wasn't always a 6XL pusher. Just nine years ago I weighed a 180-pounds, ran 10 miles a day, and eating was fuel instead of life. Not to sound like a cliché, but I was a physical force to be reckoned with. Now I'm just a physical soft-ass force that is undoubtedly physically and emotionally wrecked. Honestly, I'm not sure where I lost my way, but fast food has come to run my life. It's strange because every Monday, or 1st of the month I always tell myself "Let's change my life, watch a barrage of motivational *YouTube* videos, and promise to go on a diet that following morning."

Now my mornings usually consist of me waddling out of bed like a belly-up seal or more like a two-ton walrus trying to skirmish from one side of an iceberg to another— in this case from one side of my bed to the other. I'll immediately hit the showers, except I have to take an additional 5 to 10 more minutes than the average person, so I can make sure to lather every mass surface area. Naturally, this extra time of constant scrubbing will leave me out of breath with my hands on my knees as if I had just completed a ten-mile run for which I used to do so effortlessly almost a decade ago.

Interesting enough, on "diet days" or mostly a Monday, I'll wake-up motivated and the thought of fast food won't go further than me struggling to get out of bed, as rolling over from one side to the other will remind me of what the goal and task are for the day before I hit the showers and get ready for school. This time in my life I was going back to college, about a semester away from graduating, and unfortunately living at home with my parents at the lovely age of 32 going on 33.

Usually my morning motivation of "dieting" comes to a screeching halt by the time I instinctively look into my fridge and see an endless supply of possibilities. Predictably, I won't make breakfast because I'd much rather hit the drive-thrus and because it is a Monday, I'll drive past my neighborhood which seems to be sponsored by fast-food joints.

By the time I get to school, reflections of my glorious refrigerator will only tease my mind with ideas to please my taste buds. Also, when I drive past "fast-food alley" near my university, I've already planned a meal to pick up and take home, not to mention my lunch, dinner, and my traditional midnight onslaught of anything of the fried persuasion.

Pounding my pallet with fast-food became a daily "ritual" of sorts for me. As much as I would've loved to have had the strength to stop, and throw in a salad from time to time, I can honestly say, it never crossed my mind. Once I lost the ability to control my eating habits, it never dawned on me to ever eat healthy whenever I would go to fast-food joints. I'm not sure if it was my mind playing tricks on me, or subconsciously I was filling a "void" of sorts, but during this time in my life, I was falling and there was no way of me knowing how I could ever regain the motivation I needed to become healthy again.

# I

# THE BIRTH
## *of a junky*

# THE FALL: VOL. I

$\mathcal{W}$HEN I GRADUATED HIGH school, I weighed a 165-pound of teenage steel. I was a proud street baller, a young Don Juan, and a slacker when it came to my high school career. But this was the late 90s where being a cool slacker was socially acceptable and one could dominate the social scene by skipping school– which I was all-time great at. I would graduate in the 11th hour at the bottom 10% of my class upsetting my family. Looking back, I wish I would've taken school more seriously, so I could've had that great college experience, but unfortunately, I would enter the workforce immediately, and get punched in the face ferociously by life, nearly claiming my life, but certainly devouring my youth.

The week after my high school graduation, I met the girl of my dreams, and coincidentally began working my first job in a warehouse freezer separating chilies into bins labeled "ones, twos, and threes" for 12 hours a day. The job entailed that I freeze my ass off rummaging through an enormous pile of chilies, separating the fresh ones from the overripe ones so the distributor could send them out to different grocers depending on mileage. Despite the tough job, two weeks later it would close down leaving me to experience unemployment for the first time.

Although I lost my job, I had the pleasure of coming home to my girl Lauren. Considering that I went from girl to girl in high school, I didn't know what a "relationship" was nor understood what the concept of "love" meant until I met her. It may have been because I had "outkicked" my coverage with her flawless natural beauty, but I made sure that I did everything in my power to make Lauren happy, so I could continue being with her. Unfortunately, we only lasted a few years.

A few months after my relationship with Lauren, and upon entering my fifth job, I met another girl named Ana, who shared similar physical traits to Lauren and would last two years except our relationship would resemble a rollercoaster in the most proverbial form.

After blowing my early 20s to doomed relationships, and "Joe" jobs that did nothing to enhance my résumé. Without realizing it, I ballooned up from 165-pounds from when I graduated high school to 282-pounds by the ripe age of 23.

Strangely, for the next two years, my weight never stopped me from having a good time. I amassed maybe five more jobs in this duration all while jumping from a random girl to another without my weight ever being an issue.

I would finally attend college, but of course, flunk out by the end of the first semester only to earn a 0.3 G.P.A. Not only was I scraping the bottom of the barrel, but partying every night and having a blast until the break of dawn was becoming customary. Looking back, I do account my "flayling" in life to being a "twenty-something" and desperately searching for that "college experience" I had always craved, except without the late-night binges of studying and having my nose in a book. Instead, my late-night binges consisted of brown greased bags of stale fries and golden burger wrappers surrounding my bed like fresh mushrooms in a misty forest, or in this case in my burger. My path to 282-pounds was in every aspect unmemorable. Besides meeting new friends from my many numerous jobs, all that I ever gained was weight in the second worst possible way. I only say the "second worst possible way," because there would be many more years to come where I would implode physically wishing I would weigh 282-pounds again– unfortunately.

In retrospect, I've always heard "Never forget your past, or never have regrets; it made you who you are today." Well, for me, although the laughs and late nights were fun, I'd exchange all those *moments* for stability in my life at the time, so I'd never had to endure what I would years later, and to wear a decent size t-shirt.

*"Hi!* **WE'LL** *order your #5 six-piece chicken tender combo, but can you add two extra fried chicken strips, and make it a value meal?" I asked.*

*"…Of course, is there anything else you'd like to order, sir?" the drive-thru attendant asked.*

*"…Um…yes, can you also add a bacon breakfast sandwich!" I asked shyly.*

*"We are now offering an extra breakfast sandwich for a dollar when you order a breakfast sandwich of your choice. Would you be interested?" the drive-thru attendant asked.*

*"…Okay, make the extra one with sausage."*

# WHAT IS A DIET?

$\mathcal{I}$ WAS 282-POUNDS, HAVING A good time transitioning my new-found freedom from back to back relationships with both Lauren and Ana. Sure, while weighing three-quarters past two- hundred pounds, I was still successful with random women. In the midst of all this glory, something was missing, something was telling me that I had to fill a void of some sorts, but at the time I wasn't sure of what it was.

I was currently twenty-four years old and had flunked out of college for the second time, while also being unemployed. Eventually, I would find another job which must have been my fifteenth job, at an office supply store. Working long hours stocking and driving a fork-lift from pallet to pallet was physically taxing, and maybe what I needed to put my body through at the time, but the job was tough. The silver lining from working at this office supply store was that I would meet great friends. Now, the majority of them were all in relationships, but because they were my age or younger, they often acted single, especially in my presence. I was grateful for their company but looking back maybe we had a little too much fun as they often were getting in trouble for their angst, and hi-jinx that usually consisted of them sneaking out of their place, so they could join me at my local pub or club. This would be the job where I would meet a great friend who would eventually become my best friend by the name of Tony or Tone as I would call him. I met Tone when he was 19 years old, and we immediately hit it off. Throughout the years we would go through many war stories together. His most profound impact on me would be introducing me to the polarizing term called "diet."

As unbelievable as it sounds, I had never heard of the word "diet." Growing up in my family we ate together every night, and on my own time I'd lift weights or be at the park playing basketball. The term "diet" never crossed my path, at least to my knowledge. Looking back, I may have heard the word "diet" after all I did take health in high school and would eventually minor in kinesiology. Although I would gain my weight from when I was with both Lauren and Ana nothing was ever said about my ever-expanding waistline, because they were 5-foot-tall, weighed about a 100-pounds each, and had the ability to eat all day and never gain a single ounce.

So, when I met Tone, he would tell me this story that he had grown up in a house where his mother would always be on a diet, and often enforce it upon him during his youth, although he never had a weight issue. Naturally, Tone would grow up conscious about his weight even though he was already a good-looking guy. Tone would say that if it weren't for his short height, he would be able to maintain his physique seeing he is a fellow street baller as well, and a damn good one at that— our one on one battles, were always epic.

*×*

Three years passed, and our friendship grew to best friends. We grew so close that not only would we share deep dark secrets and goals with one another, but we also grew physically together as well, and I'm not talking about in height. I mean our waistlines grew exponentially.

So, one day Tone told me "Dude, we should diet so that we could fit into kick-ass suits." Tone at this time had a long-time girlfriend, so I knew his intention wasn't to find another girl, but because he was gaining weight, he would mention the word "diet" and educate me about it. Tone's first idea was:

"We need to cut the fatty foods, so why don't we eat only two sandwiches a day, with no chips or soda."

I was still confused by his idea, mostly because I wasn't aware that I was a fat fuck as odd as that may sound.

"Sounds good bro," I said nonchalantly.

Now, this "sandwich diet" entailed two sandwiches a day and water only. The idea being that a single sandwich couldn't be more than 300 calories, and according to dieticians we're supposed to eat 2,000 calories a day. Surely, we'd lose "CRAZY WEIGHT." Well, for two weeks we tried this diet, and we both lost fifteen pounds— we were amazed. Of course, by the end of the two weeks, we were deathly tired of sandwiches and were near a meltdown and wanted to scratch the diet altogether. That's when Tone researched and introduced me to the "low carb" diet. While Tone explained that we could eat endless meat, chicken, and fish, I was in, and couldn't wait to get started. The only catch was that we couldn't eat bread or sugar, and the term "diet" was now my every thought, and I would do anything to fit into those suits Tone had mentioned before. That night around 4:30 in the morning we'd buy an endless amount of beef so that we could transition to the "low-carb" diet in full force. Times were changing.

# BACK SEAT OF MY JEEP

 *I*N THE MIDDLE OF this "low-carb" transitional diet, I felt a bit stagnant. It was about a month after our "sandwich diet," and I had lost about 30-pounds altogether from 282- pounds to 252-pounds exactly. As for Tone, he wasn't doing too well; as a matter of fact, after the "sandwich diet" and losing those 15-pounds, he'd fallen off the wagon and gained every one of those pounds back and then some.

Naturally, after losing those quick 30-pounds, I'd plateau for about two weeks. Out of frustration, I was out of ideas. I had stayed committed to the "low-carb" diet by eating healthy proteins such as salmon, tilapia, tuna, and turkey; while also exercising by running a mile or so a day. No matter what I was doing for a two-week span, I was stuck, especially after I lost nearly a pound a day.

Then, as if God purposely threw me a lifeline knowing I was about to break and hit-up a *Whataburger* I'd get a phone call from Tone, not knowing that this phone call would change my life, perspective, or appreciation for life, I begrudgingly answered.

"What's up dawg?"

"Hey man, come outside." Tone said with optimism in his voice.

I got up from my bed and looked out my window, and saw a *Jeep* parked. Because the top was off the *Jeep*, I was able to see Tone looking up at me waving to come outside. I quickly put on my shoes and darted down the stairs to join Tone. As I turned the corner of my apartment to greet Tone, there it was: A *Jeep Wrangler*– she was gorgeous. After I greeted Tone emphatically, I couldn't help but ask.

"I didn't know you were looking for a new ride dawg?" I asked.

"Nah, it belongs to my Tio. He only has it for the night. Actually, he already sold it."

"Dang dawg this *Jeep* is pimpin, can we go for a ride?"

Although stunning, there was nothing special about the *Jeep*. No *KC* lights, snorkel or lift, but its "plain Jane" look was calling me. As the moonlight accented its fresh green paint job to resemble a metal jade, I couldn't help but tour the *Jeep* as if I was the one on the market to own such a piece of automotive perfection. I squatted down to look under the car to appear as if I knew what I was doing knowing damn well I knew shit about cars when Tone spoke.

"Hey man, let's take the doors off and go for a cruise."

I leaped up from the asphalt in sheer joy and helped Tone with the doors and put them in my apartment. Tone started the engine. The exhale from the exhaust purred from the *Jeep* resembling a moan from a hooker that met her match. I knew my world was about to change.

From my apartment Tone drove directly to the freeway. The entire way, Tone and I sat in silence as I sat there enjoying the wind hit my face while my leg stretched past where the doors would've been on top the fender of the wheel. It was a Tuesday night, so we didn't expect much traffic as we flew through the freeway like two cowboys riding through the night. As Tone took the exit towards Main Street the freedom that was pulsing through my body made me feel as if I was King of the world, and this *Jeep* was my throne.

Upon arriving at Main Street, we approached what seemed to be our first red light when suddenly a car filled with girls pulled right next to us. Although I was 252-pounds at the time, I was still confident enough to holler at any girl no matter what the situation. Seriously, we could've been in a *Pinto*, a 1988 *Buick LeSabre*, or at church and I'd say anything to an attractive girl. I stood up from the seat and held onto the windshield railing about to holler at the girls, when I noticed Tone's body language resemble a curled hermit slowly trying to hide in its shell. Tone was sinking into his chair and somehow using the stirring wheel as some kind of blocked force field from the girls. I quickly sat back into the seat in empathy.

"They ain't all that anyways dawg," I said.

"If you want to hit them up bro, go for it," Tone said.

Tone had gained some weight since the "sandwich diet" not to mention also had a long-term girlfriend, so I knew it was better if I didn't do anything to put him into such an awkward predicament. As soon as the light turned green, Tone peeled out leaving the girls to eat our dust.

It was on this ride in the *Jeep* that I felt something besides freedom. As we made our way home through the city of McAllen, I was beginning to feel rejuvenated. I began to envision being in outstanding shape driving through the town in a *Jeep* enjoying life. Although I didn't have a *Jeep*, I knew that if I got to my goal of weighing a 180-pounds than not only would I be physically happy, but I'd rule the world.

Images flashed through my mind of me driving through town with the wind in my hair and a dime piece by my side all while LL Cool J's "*Back Seat of my Jeep*" played off my 18-inch *Rockford Frostgate* speakers. Another image came to me, except this one was of Lauren and me in the back seat of my *Jeep* and instead of the famed lyric from LL's song "extensions on the carpet," it would be Lauren and me on the *Jeep's* carpet fully engaged from what used to be.

After Tone dropped me off, I couldn't sleep a wink and would decide to go for a run well past midnight. Except I was so full of adrenaline, and instead of running my one to two miles this night would be the first time I'd run five miles non-stop, and to be honest I sincerely felt as if I could've ran another five. After my second shower of the night, I was still full of energy and decided to call into work, so I could spend the day exercising to reach my weight loss goal sooner rather than later.

Three months later, I would reach 180-pounds. In the months after that fateful night with Tone and the *Jeep,* I was still motivated. After I ran those five miles that now became the baseline for every run I did every single one of those days. There was even a point where on the weekends when I was off from work that I'd run ten to twelve miles all while eating insanely light. By this time, I was only eating egg whites for breakfast, a small can of tuna for lunch, and for dinner, I'd go even lighter and eat another can of tuna surely hitting Ketosis which is when your body uses your stored fat for energy. I'm not sure if it was a three-month adrenaline bomb, but those visions of me experiencing those fantasies in that *Jeep* was ALL I wanted, and I was finally there.

# THE GOOD LIFE

*I* WAS NEW, I WAS spry, and most importantly I could fit into a large t-shirt with change. Granted, this was 2006/2007, and those times were different from now. Almost eight years later I'd be weighing a full-on 401-pound, but I digress.

Sadly for Tone, he would continue to struggle with his weight. I suppose that night in the *Jeep* wasn't as inspiring for him as it was for me. As for Tone, his Everest was getting under a 198-pounds, as it seemed every time he'd hit the 198-pound marker, he would fall off the wagon time and time again. According to Tone, his downfall was his tortured relationship with his then-girlfriend Francis. Tone would eventually balloon up to 256-pounds and believe me when I say this. When you are 5'7 and weigh 256-pounds, you might as well be 5'11 and weigh 300-pounds like I eventually would. Because of Tone's tumultuous relationship with his bitch of a girlfriend, I believed she feared my phoenix-like ascension towards the heavens thinking I'd influence Tone to a binge of booze, bitches, and "mota" which is Spanish slang for weed or what we had nicknamed it "Wooly Mammoth." Was Tone's girl right about her assumption of me? Of course, but the times it did occur were rare, leaving Tone to be a spectator to all my events. The main question I would ask though was "Did she have to fatten him up to the point where he'd waddle to the restroom just to take a piss?"

Now, at the time I was living with a friend of a friend who needed a roommate, and she was quintessentially the greatest most bonafide dime-piece I've ever seen by the name of Olivia. She was five years my senior, but unfortunately, I was placed in a worse category than the dreaded "friend zone." Instead, I was put into the "little brother" category even when I was in shape. She would introduce me to her friends as her "little brother" as well. Safe to say nothing ever happened.

At this phase of my life, I was running 8-12 miles a day, while eating nothing but "low carb" anything, all while kicking life's ass. I made it a point that I'd isolate myself until I hit a 180-pounds exactly. If I came in at 181-pounds or even a single pound over, I committed to isolation. It was a promise to myself that the day I was 180 would be the day I'd live forever.

*** 

It was October 31, Halloween. I was 25 at the time, and because of a traumatic experience in 7th grade, I never dressed up, much less thought it was stupid as fuck. That morning I felt my stomach was flat and empty, probably because the night before I ran my record 15 miles and spent that night shitting anacondas. I approached the scale like a hungry boxer ready to take on the champ about to weigh in. As I stepped upon my old school off-white scale, the dial spun like a D.J. scratching a record. I looked down in deep anticipation. Upon opening my squinted eyes, I saw the scale read a 178-pounds. I hunched over to double check and to make certain the lining of the scale was accurate— it seemed a half pound off. I stepped off to readjust the motherfucker only to step on it again this time with my eyes pierced upon the scale. It read 179. I shouted out to the heavens "BOOM-BAP!" I immediately called Tone who at the time I hadn't seen since that glorious night with the *Jeep* to tell him the great news.

"What up motherfucka!" I said to an exhausted Tone.

"Shit, chillin dawg, what's up?" Tone said.

"Dawg! You and I let's hit the club." I asked with deep anticipation.

"I don't know dude; I'd have to check with the boss," Tone said disappointedly.

"Come on man, tell her you're going to play basketball like back in the days when I always kicked your ass," I said emphatically.

"Let me see what I can do; I'll hit you up later."

"Tell her you're going to get some exercise, I'm sure she'll be down with that," I said.

I would also text message my childhood homeboys Alejandro, Chuck (who we called Chuco,) and Nick. I grew up with all of them, and they had grown to like Tone very much even to the point where they would go out without me at times, which I'll admit bothered me at first, but after everything Tone had gone through, I'm happy he'd found solace in my homies.

Now, living in McAllen, Texas you were either going to school to become a teacher (which I eventually would,) become a border patrol agent (ironically,) or work the oil fields as did Alejandro, Chuco, and eventually Tone. As for Nick, he went back to school also to become an educator.

Instead of waiting for their replies, I would walk over to my closet. One side of my closet was my transitioning clothes from the 3XL all the way to XL. Before today, I always rocked my XLs at work even though they draped over me like an obese southern red neck woman wearing a tired out moomu. On the other side of the closet was my new fresh clothing I hadn't worn and was waiting to wear for such an occasion. My clothes varied from collared button-up shirts, fitted *Polo's*, and t-shirts with various artists such *as: Biggie Smalls* Album *Ready to Die, Bob Marley, Metallica's Ride the Lightning,* and my favorite t-shirt which was an abstract portrait of my hero/homeboy Cesar Chavez with detailed skull faces of farm workers and their protest constructing a portrait of Cesar Chavez's face.

For tonight, I decided to keep it simple: Fresh socks, fresh dark jeans, fresh black boxer briefs, a fresh solid black t-shirt, and new fresh white *Air Force Ones.* Dressed, I would bring the unopened orange *Nike box,* and sit on the side of my made bed. I slowly opened the box as if I was about to open a detonator of sorts delicately. There they were sitting in all its magnificent clean glory. Size: 10.5 *Air Force Ones.* I lifted the left shoe and instinctively breathed in its fresh new sole and grinned as I'm sure I resembled a mother smelling her newborn baby for the first time. I scanned each sneaker making sure it hadn't been tampered with— they were pristine.

I felt like I was in a ritual getting assembled as a new 179-pound man. I recalled an old homie of mine and his crew living and dying by a "ritual" as part of their mantra, as I got dressed in this version of their "ritual." After I slicked back my hair, I knew I was ready to commence and shift the world, and most importantly get laid, which unfortunately was about to hit the one-year mark.

I checked my phone, and my boys were all down and excited to go. Thankfully both Alejandro, and Chuco were here on break from the oil rigs. As for Tone, he hadn't been working the rigs yet but was home the entire summer in which we hadn't spoken to one another since. I could only assume he had been trying to work things out with Francis.

\*\*\*

I arrived at *Luka bar* a few minutes before I wanted to, but I was here and ready for my first appearance in years. I approached the club/bar like a gladiator approaching the Roman Coliseum. I felt nervous, but for some strange reason my confidence obliterated my nerves, and I knew it was because for the first time in months I was walking freely without the physical pains that comes from being a large man.

It was like I walked into a grand party— something of which Marie Antoinette would approve. Dime pieces were everywhere, and they were looking at me like I was the Hope diamond. I smirked knowing without a doubt in my mind that my drought was about to be over, and I couldn't wait. Suddenly, I would hear someone shout my name.

"Tre!"

I turned to look, and sure enough, it was my homeboys accompanied by stunning women I had never met before.

*"Did they pick them up here?"* I thought.

*Who gives a fuck?* Their faces were joyous as their smiles extended from exit to exit, surprised to see how fantastic I looked— which I must admit, I looked and felt like a male version of a dime piece, a modern Mexican replica of the statue of David, but more adequately proportioned to my body; especially now— that poor bastard.

After countless compliments, I realized everyone had someone to be with but me. They all looked happy as we sat in the corner of the club— the girls on one side and us fellas on the other except Tone who of course was sitting in the middle next to his girl looking miserable. For me, I was alone for sure. I surveyed the dance floor and realized *"Oh fuck!"* I haven't danced in years, and since I had always claimed myself an old soul because of my love for Jazz, old sports statistics, and literature of the "Lost Generation;" the dancing I was accustomed to was 90s hip-hop (bump & grind) edition. Was I the best at it? Of course not, but I could certainly move and groove to the beat without hesitation— especially now that I had this new-found flexibility.

I couldn't wait to expose my "dirty eagle" dance that I had stolen from Tone. A dance move he had perfected that had all the power in the world to make all the panties on the dance floor fall off with extra bounce. I know I'm exaggerating, but with this newfound confidence and body, I felt like Adonis would bow down to me.

I decided to strut to the dance floor and approach the first dime I see.

"Hey, you want to dance?" I said maybe a little too eagerly.

"Um. Sorry, I'm dancing with my girlfriend," she said after looking me up and down as if I was under evaluation.

*"0 for 1,"* I thought.

I approached another girl. This time a five-footer.

"Hey, you want to dance? I asked while shimmying my shoulders like a dumbass to the beat.

"No, I'm sorry my boyfriend is buying me a drink," she said.

"Cool, cool," I said.

I walked away certainly conscious of "the walk of shame." Now I felt a surge of sympathy I used to give all my old random one nighters back in the days.

The night continued, and I was 0 for 7. *Holy shit!* I thought. Maybe I wasn't ready to be here; maybe I needed to lose another 10-pounds. *SHIT!*

I began second guessing myself. I turned to look at my boys. I noticed Chuco getting a "rub job" while watching me swing and miss. Tone seemed to be apologizing for something he probably never did— Jesus fuck! Francis must give great head for him to put up with her bullshit. As for Alejandro, he was in a current make-out session, and if I'm not mistaken it appeared he might have switched girls with Nick who was currently in a make-out session as well with whom I presumed was Alejandro's girl, or whatever.

I turned back to the dance floor feeling an enormous amount of pressure. I noticed in the far corner a group of five girls all who seemed deep into some lame conversation, except the girl on the end appearing bored, maybe the younger sister who was forced into coming along— I could only pray. *"Should I throw her a bone?"* I thought. I mean how sweet would it be if I approached her, and asked her to dance? She would without a doubt be the envy of her sister and friends. She wasn't the finest of the group, her wavy dark hair cascading along her dainty shoulders while hardly wearing any make-up— she surely was a natural beauty. She was in no way a dud. I quickly bought a beer. My theory was that by holding a beer, it provides somewhat of a comforting anchor, so I wouldn't look like a dumbass talking to a girl, and not knowing what to do with my hands. I strutted over to the girl, a strut that would make the intro from *Saturday Night Fever* seem weak. The closer I approached her, I began to think that she might be closer to a dime piece than I thought. I tapped her from behind her shoulder.

"Hey what's up? I'm Tre, I want to ask if I can buy you a drink?"

I asked not sure if I didn't look too desperate. I noticed her friends looked at me like "Why is he talking to her, and not me?" As each one of them looked me up and down. I smiled through their evaluation making sure my dimples dotted the exclamation point to their assessment, all while luring her in.

"Um... sure," she said.

*"Holy shit!"* I thought.

"Cool, and your name?" I asked.

"Rosie."

"Hi, Rosie."

We both walked to the bar, and she ordered a *Smirnoff* bottle leading me to believe she was not a big drinker or much of a beer drinker. We both approached the dance floor, and thankfully 90s hip-hop was on. It was like we were in sync while dancing. When I went down, she went down. When I moved left, she went left— it was beautifully rhythmic and sexy. I placed my hand on her waist and pulled her in— the Holy Ghost had no chance. We locked eyes, and I just went for it. Without resistance, we fully embraced. My kissing drought was officially over. Thoughts of my last make-out session flashed in my mind, and I couldn't help but grin as our tongues tumbled over one another. Then like a bolt of lightning, it hit me. *How do I transition and take her home to end another streak?* Suddenly, my mind whispered to me "Come on Tre, you've been waiting for this your whole life. Be the old Tre." Strangely, I nodded confidently while making-out with Rosie, and visualized the great Tim Duncan locking down Kevin Garnett— I suddenly knew what to do.

The song finally finished, and by this time small talk had remained at large. I decided to keep it simple, and whisper in her ear.

"I don't live too far away," I said smoothly.

I smiled as she smiled. Suddenly, Montel Jordan's *"This Is How We Do It"* went from its rhythmic funk sound to a muffled tone-def ring as I was sure my newly thinned out faced had some desperate, hopeful expression.

"Let's go," she said.

It was as if I just scored the winning touchdown, and the University of Texas Longhorns fight song played in my head. Ba, ba, baaa, ba, ba, baaa, ba, ba ba baa ba ba ba baaa. I pulled her by the hand and saluted Tone, Nick, and the fellas as they saluted me back in grand fashion. I exited the club with my index finger wagging in the air reminiscent of Joe Namath's walk-off.

***

Nights like this would become a regular for me. Closing home loans at work was more difficult than picking up women— Jesus fuck! Life was good for the next year, year and a half. At the end of the day, as great as it was to pick-up women, feeling great, running 10 miles a day, and living the good life, eventually, that would all come to a screeching halt as the all mighty burger would become far more important for years to come.

# THE POP-IN

*J* MAY HAVE EXPERIENCED THE "good life" for about 16 months. The last four of those months was when the wheels started to fall off the fucking hinges. Now, I was still getting laid on a near daily basis with random women, but something was entering my mind while in a "bang session" with some dime piece, which were thoughts of *Whataburger*. I mean seriously, an image of a #2 combo from *Whataburger* would replace the face of the underlying girl. Instead of going in for a kiss, I would seriously envision a #2 double meat *Whataburger* with cheese. Silly? Maybe, but that was the damn truth.

About a year and a half after that infamous night at *Luka bar* when I finally weighed a 179-pounds, I had ballooned up to 217-pounds. A near 40-pound influx of saturation. At this time, I experienced a damn right embarrassing moment for me, and that was when Tone popped into my apartment. Unbeknownst to Tone, at the time I was going through an insane binge of the critically acclaimed *HBO* TV series *Sopranos*, and this was way before TV binges became the cliché that they have become now— so, I'd like to take the credit for that, but I digress.

The day Tone walked into my apartment, and eventually to my bedroom, changed everything for me from an embarrassing standpoint. I tried my best to hold Tone in my living room to have a beer or two, but because of my lack of furniture in my apartment, my bedroom would call naturally as it was the only room with a television and an extra seat. Upon entering my bedroom, I knew I was in for a rude awakening, and Tone was about to experience the ugly side of addiction that one day he'd be all too familiar with as well, so why not introduce him to his near future. Not even a step in and Tone would stop dead in his tracks and witness a cluster fuck of *Whataburger* bags, golden cheeseburger wrappers, and 32-ounce Styrofoam cups surrounding my bed rivaling anything that had ever been seen on another acclaimed TV show called *Hoarders*. I'll never forget Tone's facial expression or reaction which completely detailed shock and awe in the most natural of ways.

"Dude, I can't even see your tile floor bro," Tone said.

"Um, wait," I said.

"Are you okay? Are you not running anymore?" Tone asked.

Until today I hadn't seen Tone in a few months, so I'm sure he noticed my obvious weight gain.

"Nah duke! I'm just on this crazy ass *Soprano* binge," I said.

"You've already seen that series like three times dawg," Tone said while still trying to process what was going on in my room.

"I know man, but the show teaches you something new every time," I said.

The judgment stopped there as Tone would join me in a 3-episode binge that night, along with a full course of *Whataburger*. When the last episode concluded, a 2-hour long discussion about the many life lessons from *The Sopranos* occurred; that's when he and I came up with an idea.

"Dude, we should move in together, imagine all the pirated shit we could watch? Shit would be dope," Tone said.

Tone had made a living cleaning computers and selling pirated videos, so the offer was intriguing.

"You serious?" I said.

"Fuck yeah bro!" Tone said.

"What about your boss?" I said referring to Francis.

"She'll chill with me, but she won't be living with us."

I knew Tone was bull-shittin about his girl, but because he has always had "pussy on a pedestal," I'm sure she'd be a third roommate.

I thought of my roommate Olivia and considered her unparalleled beauty, and how I'd miss seeing her perfect mug. She was always the perfect visualization for when I wanted to extend the night with a random girl— along with a *Whataburger* of course.

"I don't know man; I'll miss Olivia," I said.

"Please, you said it yourself that you hate it when she refers to you as her little brother."

Hearing Tone utter the phrase "little brother," only confirmed that no such occurrence would ever happen to where I could ever seal the deal with Olivia.

"Alright my man, I'm in."

"Not only can we binge on movies, but we can start working out together and get cheese." Tone said.

The term "cheese," was our silly way of saying getting into shape.

That weekend Francis, Tone, and I settled into our new apartment. It was nothing impressive; it was a standard two-bedroom, two-bath white tile and white cabinet little joint. Of course, because Tone and Francis were together, they occupied the much larger room with a restroom— fucking ass-hole.

The first day Tone and I moved in we both stepped onto a scale to measure the first night living together in hopes that it be a measuring date to when we hit our weight loss goal— once again. Tone would weigh in at 256, while I came in at 217-pounds. We were both stunned. My solution to this was to begin playing basketball. Our apartment was close to a basketball court, so a walk over to play and a walk back would surely have us lose weight in no time. As for Tone, he was so devastated by his weigh-in, and wouldn't say much. He just mumbled under his breath "I'll figure it out. Damn!" and head right into his room ending a short night on move-in day.

That night I would lace up my *Jordan 11* Space Jams, and head out to the park. Now the walk was longer than I thought, but the court was empty thankfully. I would spend about an hour getting my 3-point shot back and knock down as many free throws in a row as possible— most was 17. I didn't produce as much sweat as I'd like, but I was moving, which was something I hadn't done in months. At least it was a good start, and a change from that day Tone had seen my bedroom littered with "greased debris." I came home to Tone blasting some dumbass house music that was rattling the walls. My picture frame that was a gift had taken a hard spill causing me to think that I may have made a mistake moving in.

# FAST-FOOD ALLEY

*O*VER THE NEXT FEW weeks, I would grow immune to the house music and learn to sleep with it blasting throughout the apartment. Another aspect that I became accustomed to was the numerous fast food joints that surrounded our neighborhood. The tall neon signs that rivaled the Vegas strip made it impossible to continue playing basketball only to hit the fast food restaurants and go "ham" on hamburgers instead. For a fast food junky, it became even more impossible to resist a midnight splurge that would be anyone else's entire week of junk food, and for me, it was "late dinner."

Another aspect of being a junky is getting someone else to do junk with, and of course, I'd have Tone hitch onto my glorious downfall. Predictably, our apartment began to resemble my old bedroom from when I lived with Olivia except it wasn't just *Whataburger* wrappers, and Styrofoam cups. Because of Tone's exotic pallet, our rooms, and living room became layered with pizza boxes, Chinese, and Tex-Mex botana platters which consisted of refried beans and melted cheddar cheese on tortilla chips topped with beef and chicken fajita. If we wanted to be healthy about the botana platter, we'd substitute the beef and chicken fajita with mariscos (seafood) — it was deliciously horrendous.

After this barrage of junk food, this would be the beginning of a new drought. Since I lost the weight the first time; the longest I ever went without a piece of ass was maybe two to three weeks, and now I was about to experience true sexual *deprivity* for the first time since *Luka Bar.*

The strip of junk food lights glittered along the infamous street that could be viewed from the space station. The fast-food strip was too much for me to deny completely, compromising my desire I ever had for pussy, leaving me to get to know my hand embarrassingly. Jesus, I wish I had pussy on a pedestal.

Eventually, Tone's girl left him, and even though she claimed "she fell out of love" we both knew it was because of Tone's husky frame. Tone and I lived together for two more years. Tone gained about five more pounds which would catch him by surprise considering how hard we hit that fast food strip every day. As for me, I went from 217 to a booming 265-pounds.

The fast-food strip would soon be renamed "Fast-Food Alley," and shame and embarrassment would occupy us both as weekends turned into gluttonous binges of grease and hacked movies only to conclude with a vacant bed surrounded by shame.

# PRIORITIES

$\mathcal{A}$ FEW WEEKS INTO LIVING with Tone, we had both fallen into a predictable path of gluttony and slothery. Were we at the time aware of our tag-team version of deadly sins? Yes! We were, and to be honest; we were having a great time. There were days where movement may have consisted of body scratching only. If *Fitbits* were around back then, I'm more than sure we'd total a hundred steps combined.

Although, I was aware of my recent weight gain, I was still hooking up with girls, except not at the rapid pace from when I was a 180-pounds. During this duration, I was talking to a girl named Julie who was a past "random," and at times a repeat customer, but it had been a while. Because I had been on my longest sex drought since I was a 180-pounds, I knew I had to put an end to such blasphemy, so predictably I called Julie, not because she was a repeat customer, but because she was fantastic in the sack. While eating in abundance with our guts inflated pointed directly to the ceiling, I had been texting with Julie non-stop discussing everything from our favorite books *(Post Office)* for me, to her promiscuity from being a virgin until she was 20 and then spending the next 5 years trying to hit the "centennial marker" for hooking up with random men. I will admit that if I looked at her as more than another "notch" on my belt than her promiscuity would've certainly bothered me, but in the most selfish of ways, I just wanted to end my drought.

I had also noticed during this period that Francis hadn't come by, and my often glutton fests had been more of a solo job often binge eating 3-4 times a day certainly passing the 10,000-calorie mark. One day Tone knocked on my door to ask if I wanted to join him in eating at *Jack-In-The-Box*. At the time *Jack-in-the-Box* had become our main source of shame, and if I was not mistaken this was the second time *Jack-in-the-Box* then appropriately nicknamed (JIB-U) as in *Jack-in-the-Box* University had been my focus of shame. I would learn on the way to JIB-U that Tone and Francis had been on a week break. Immediately, I was filled with happiness due to my disdain for Francis, but I could tell by Tone's voice that he was a bit distraught. I would inform Tone about Julie to change the subject, but his obsession with what Francis may have been doing during their time apart had overwhelmed him. I'd learn that Francis had grown tired of Tone's lazy antics and that she needed a break, or as she phrased it "I need time to miss you," which I knew meant that she was tired of Tone's ass, and knew that their relationship was ticking, I just hoped Tone knew what to expect so he wouldn't be as hurt. While waiting in the drive-thru from JIB-U, a brief silence from Tone would be interrupted when I'd see two attractive girls walk by my car, one resembling Julie, and that's when our silence was broken, and I had a thought.

"Listen man, I'm going to have Julie come by this weekend, why don't I ask her to bring a friend and I'll get you laid," I said.

"No, that's okay, I'm sure Francis and I will patch things up eventually. Besides, I don't think I have the power to keep such a secret from her; she could sniff that out in a hurry."

"Come on man, when was the last time you were with her?" I asked.

I knew I wasn't being a good supportive friend, but in all honesty, I had never seen Tone and me together as a tandem.

"Nah, I'm good." Tone said.

My eyes followed both girls into JIB-U.

"Dude, has she called you at least?" I asked.

"Nope, not a single time."

"Then I hate to say this, but she's probably talking to some other dude."

Tone dips his head into his palms frustrated emotionally.

"I'm sure she isn't man, I'm messin with you. Listen, why don't we have a poker night, and if things get uncomfortable I'll call it off, I just need you there to be a buffer, and if Francis calls you in that time, I promise I'll call the whole thing off, so you won't feel guilty what-so-ever."

"I don't know, knowing my luck Francis would probably "pop-in" during our poker game, and the shit would hit the fan."

"At least you'd know you'd get laid."

"You can't guarantee that." Tone said.

"I'm sure if I tell Julie to find someone who's willing, then she'd certainly come through," I said.

"I don't know; I'd have to think about it." Tone said.

That night after our engorgement of JIB-U and a pirated movie, I was able to convince Tone to join Julie and me for a poker night, which Julie would later message me stating that she knew the perfect girl for Tone considering she had never met him. My new goal besides ending my drought was now getting Tone laid at whatever the cost—challenge excepted.

***

The night before our poker night, Tone and I cleaned up our apartment using about 5 or 6 *Hefty* bags to pick up our abundance of food sponsored from fast food alley. Everything from Chinese and Mexican platters to my clichéd mountain-sized golden wrappers from burger joints along with numerous 32 to 48-ounce Styrofoam soft drinks. All though I was still able to fit into my old clothing at the time, I would've not been surprised in the few weeks since I had moved in that we may have gained about 20 pounds each, but as long as the shirts were fitting, then there would be nothing to worry about.

The night of our poker game, I advised Tone to call or text message Francis just for safe keeping. The last thing I wanted was for us to be getting into a game of poker and suddenly Francis pop-in and start all this hell only confirming what Tone had feared. Tone would call Francis, and she'd never answer; Tone would leave her a voicemail and a text message and predictably she never responded. After Julie messaged me that they were on their way to our place, Tone had stayed locked in his room for which I could only assume he was waiting to hear anything from Francis. Before I'd knock on his door to tell him that Julie and her friend were on their way, I'd look to see if there was any light beaming from under his door and it was pitch black. I'd also put my ear to his door, and there was no sound, as a matter of fact, you could hear the winds from his ceiling fan pulse through the door. *Shit!* I whispered under my breath; I was beginning to worry if Tone was going to leave me stranded, then predictably thoughts *of maybe I could close both girls and seriously end my drought in the GREATEST of ways.* Then I was reminded that if Francis was going to punk Tone, then I had to put my greed aside and get Tone laid at whatever the cost. I grazed Tone's door barely knocking when Tone opened his door with gusto and walked past me appearing pissed but in a strange way like a man on a mission.

"What's up? You alright?" I asked.

"I'm good bro, when is your friend coming by."

I smiled delightedly to finally experience what life would be like with me and Tone single for the first time. This poker night was years in the making, and we were ready to take on the world.

As Tone got dressed, I was setting up the poker chips and table when suddenly the doorbell rang. I smiled sinisterly and instantly knew that it was SHOWTIME. I put the chips down and called Tone who was looking fresh, and sharp as ever at least for a 260-pounder. Looking back, I would currently kill to look 260-pounds, as Tone did then. It was game-time, and although we were both fat fuckers, I embraced this current shift of magnitude Tone and I were experiencing, I even enjoyed the walk to the door envisioning a slow-motion strut you'd see from the movies—I was in love with this moment.

I'd open the door, and Julie looked stunning as did her friend, for which she looked familiar. I turned my head like a dog confused because I knew I knew her from somewhere from my past. I'd see her eyes swell with worry and awkwardness when Julie introduced us.

"Hey Tre, this is my friend Brandy."

As I shook her hand and introduced Tone, it suddenly hit me that Brandy was one of my first "randoms" after that legendary night at *Luka* Bar. I wanted to pull Tone aside and give him the news, but the way he was looking at her and Julie made me realize that whatever happened this night would certainly be one for the books and the Tre-N-Tone Experience or the T-N-T Experience was about to commence.

After a quick tour of our apartment Tone shyly lagged, it was clear he was out of his element, and to be honest, I couldn't blame him. I mean it had been years since he was single, so I knew that it would take a while for him to get comfortable with Brandy who by the way was walking closer to me than Julie ever was especially when I showed them my bedroom. Tone's awkward shyness as he lagged behind the tour was beginning to make me uncomfortable, and to be honest, I wanted to pull in Julie for a quick "session" before our poker night began, but there was no way Tone would have known what to do with Brandy. I would have had better odds commencing in a 3-way than Tone "sealing the deal." Instead, I cut the tour short and led everyone to the poker table so we could all become acclimated with one another, and most importantly get Tone comfortable.

After passing everyone nice cold beers, I suggested that we play Texas Hold'em when Tone shouts.

"No way man, you'd kill us, and this game would be over in ten minutes."

During this duration of time, Texas Hold'em had become the next hot thing in sports coverage; especially in my household. As for me, I had gotten pretty good even to the point where I hooked up with a random girl all because I beat the table handily concluding the night with a spectacular ending fit to be seen on *ESPN* top 10 highlights.

"Come on, it's an easy game to understand, and it's fun," I said

"Yeah, I've heard you're pretty good. I want to see you in action." Brandy said as she slid her hand on my shoulder. I smiled slightly looking over to Tone and Julie making sure they never noticed the obvious flirting being done by Brandy risking my night with Julie. Thankfully both Julie and Tone were both too busy counting their chips. "Okay, let's get started," I said.

After a few hands in we were more immersed in conversation about Julie's new-found promiscuity than the actual poker game. If I remembered correctly, I hadn't won a single hand, I was just fascinated by the fact that Julie's quest to break the centennial mark with men was real, and somewhat proud that I was on that list not to mention the fact that I was a "repeat customer" which filled me with pride that I was able to satisfy her enough to keep her coming back considering her conquest. Of course, the counter-argument was Tone mentioning that, because she was beautiful, reaching her "centennial mark" should be easy because she's an attractive girl. That if she wanted to, she could sleep with a different man a day if she so desired to. Naturally, we'd all agree with Tone's assessment of her conquest, but Julie made her mission clear that she'd never pursue, that it was up to the man to "close her," or as she put it "I'm old fashioned like that" which of course brought hilarity to our poker game. We'd also learn that Brandy was a devout virgin through most of her years in high school because of her religion, but when she met a much older man, even as a 17-year-old she couldn't resist. Then mentions the day she went to college was like unleashing her to the wolves claiming college may have led her to become a sex addict. Which was obvious because of our past, and by the way she was looking at me. I looked over to Tone, and I could tell that he was finally relaxed. Hearing the tales of both Julie and Brandy's experiences was enough to shatter any kind of discomfort and shyness from anyone much less Tone.

Considering the night began around 8 p.m. It was well past 2 a.m., and I was playing surprisingly bad. We'd also take breaks to dance whenever a great club song played over my then stereo system having a blast. Tone would loosen up exposing his legendary "dirty eagle" dance to both Julie and Brandy making it evident that he also wanted to get laid—I was so proud of him. Eventually, we'd get back to playing poker, now with Brandy leaning closer to Tone and often sliding her hand up and down his shoulder and knee, it was clear the "T-N-T Experience" was indeed gaining traction, and often distracting me from my poker hands. I'd envision how both Tone and I would rule the world, and perhaps join Julie in her endeavor of sleeping with a hundred different men, except for us, it'd be women.

Julie began telling her story of the "best man" she had ever slept with, and although I'd hope it was about me, it wasn't. But because she had a way of putting humor into her stories, the fact that she wasn't talking about me didn't faze me in the least. Julie emphasized that the man wasn't the most physically adequate man she had ever been with, but he was by far the most "giving" even to the point where she'd be willing to put on pause her "Centennial run" because of his generosity. Of course, hilarity would ensue when suddenly Brandy had to excuse herself from the table to take a phone call outside. As Julie went on and on about him, I believe I had won my first hand in a while, and without realizing Tone had a huge pile of chips followed by Julie, me then Brandy. I began to think that Julie was using her fascinating stories to distract me, which sadly worked if that was her intention. About ten minutes passed when Brandy comes in a hurry grabbing her purse and jacket stating that she had to go because it was getting late. I looked over to Tone, and I could see the instant disappointment as Brandy seemed to have rushed out the apartment without ever acknowledging her desire for Tone while also never saying "good-bye," she just rushed out. I whispered "damn-it" to myself in frustration. Julie walked Brandy outside leading me to believe that Julie would have to leave also because they came in one car making the night become a "bust." I knew I had to say something to Tone.

"It's alright my man, you win some, and you lose some, that's the nature of the beast."

Tone nods as he shuffles the deck disappointingly.

Suddenly, Julie closes the door and sits back down comfortably.

"You ready bitches!"

"I thought you were going too? Didn't you come in one car?" I said confused.

"No, we both came in our separate cars. Brandy's boyfriend is a bartender, and he just got out of work."

Tone looked over at me upset, as I shrugged my shoulders to perceive that I didn't know she had a boyfriend because I honestly didn't.

"I thought you said she was single?" I asked.

"I thought they broke up; they're always fighting," Julie said.

"Well, that's fucked up," I said as I leaned back in my chair upset.

"I'm sorry Tone, I'm sure they'll fight again, and she'd call you," Julie said somewhat sarcastically.

"Fuck that! Don't give her the time of day she doesn't deserve you!" I said.

"Yeah, she is not girlfriend material Tone, she'd use you up and spit you out especially because you're such a nice guy," Julie said.

I could tell that Tone was upset but appeared somewhat relieved; perhaps he wasn't ready for the "T-N-T Experience" to ever commence. Considering, we had a great night, and at times I felt Tone was going to close Brandy, maybe the world and I weren't ready for such an experience as well.

"It's all good, I have a girlfriend also, and even though she's on a date with some other cocksucka, I suppose my time will come."

Tone's reveal took me by total surprise. I had no idea that my prediction of Francis being with another guy was real. No wonder Tone had let loose when both Julie and Brandy showed up to our apartment. Tone would deal the cards when both Julie and I sat in silence due to Tone's revealing awkwardness. I was the small blind from our 5-10 game; I had a Jacks of diamonds and a One-Eyed Jack of hearts. My eyes swelled with optimism as I tried to hide my "tell" deceptively. It was up to Tone to call, raise or fold as he doubles the blind. "Shit," Julie says under her breath as she slouches down, tossing her cards towards the center of the table.

"What? You're doing well and can afford to at least see the flop. Besides you're the big blind." Tone said appearing somewhat determined and inspired.

"Okay, I guess you're right," Julie said disappointingly matching Tone's raise.

After I called and met the big blind, Tone draws the three cards. The first being a 7 of hearts, a 5 of hearts, and then a Jack of clubs, I desperately tried to resist grinning, because I knew this game was a wrap unless Tone had the other Jack. Julie slouches down in her chair once again "What the fuck?" and tosses her cards onto the center of the table even before I could set my bet. I wanted to see if Tone had the other Jack and built the pot, so instead of raising a large sum, I decided to keep it modest and put in $20 worth of chips. Julie was out when Tone quickly decides to raise my $20 and puts in a $100.

"What? You got a pair of jacks' cocksucka?!" I said.

"Are you going to call or run like a bitch." Tone said.

I smiled as Julie sat up intrigued.

"Fine, I'll call. This is stupid, so early in the game." I said.

Tone burns the card and turns—It's a 3 of diamonds.

"Ahh man, I had a 3," Julie said.

"Thank you for the reveal." Tone said.

I must admit that I took Julie's reveal the same way. Either Tone had the other Jack or is playing for the straight flush or flush as was I. It was my turn to bet, and because Tone was already calling me names, I couldn't let him faze me, and risk going all in. Besides, I wanted to bait him a little bit more. I put in $200 worth of chips. Tone calls and tosses in a $500 chip like he was tossing a penny into a fountain. I chuckle out loud thinking Tone was trying to play me for a fool, so I called his raise waiting for the River. Tone burns the top card and turns the river card ever so slowly. It's the One-Eyed Jack of spades. I wanted to lean back in victory but decided to not budge a single inch from my body. Julie shouts out loud. "Holy shit! Theirs's a pair of jacks! Either someone has a three or four-of-a-kind, or someone is bullshittin." Obviously, Tone had nothing. The best he was hoping for was a flush, but that 3 of diamonds fucked him up. I knew Tone was beaten, and I could go all in, but I knew if I did Tone would fold, so instead, I put in another $500 worth of chips. Tone begins to count his chips; now I was beginning to see that this hand was all about ego. *Did he need to win this hand?* I thought. I noticed Julie now flirting with Tone, perhaps to increase her number as she may have been attracted to his assertiveness from this hand. I smiled thinking *I promised to get him laid anyways.* Julie wraps her arm through Tone's arm and places her head on his shoulder, as he counts his chips.

"I'll buy all your chips." Tone said with confidence.

I looked back at my cards barely lifting them off the table. I see Tone put his head on Julie's trying to play off his bluff when I gathered all my chips and thought *should I go all in?* The way Julie was attached to Tone, it'd be a shame if I crushed him most likely leading Julie to pull away from him, so she could be with a real hero. I'd put both my hands on the base of my chips to put-in, when I'd see Julie squeeze Tone's arm even tighter. As Tone looked at me with hollowed intensity, I grinned slightly and decided to fold instead. Tone and Julie jump up from the table as if they had just won the World Series of Poker. As they danced around me, I was happy for Tone. I'm not sure if it was my right to give him such a feeling at all, but I knew he needed some kind of victory. With the sudden departure of Brandy and the revealing of Francis, I knew any new feeling no matter how small was necessary for Tone at this exact moment.

Tone had a commanding lead, and we may have played two more hands when Julie asked.

"Is it cool if I stay the night? It's late; I've had a lot to drink and don't want to drive home this late."

I looked over to Tone, and he knew this was his moment to "close" Julie and said. "Of course, you can sleep in my bed, no problem."

"No, no, I'll sleep on your couch," Julie said.

"It's no big deal really; I love that couch." Tone said.

"Are we done playing poker?" I asked.

"Yeah, I'm "pokered" out. You guys finish if you want to." Julie said.

"Yeah man, if you want to keep playing let's do it." Tone said with arrogance.

There was a small part of me that wanted to take back what I gave Tone, but I knew if Julie fell asleep on that couch while Tone and I played poker, then my promise to Tone would fall through.

"Nah, I'm good bro, I'm tired. Congrats on your winnings you can buy yourself something from fast food alley if you want." I said.

"Cool, cool. Julie, let me get you a pillow and blanket." Tone said.

As Julie laid on the couch, I looked over to Tone and winked to him signaling for him to close the deal. Tone would slightly smirk in response, as I presumed that he would be able to end the night on a great note.

Before I crashed onto my bed, I put on some music so if Tone indeed "sealed the deal" with Julie, I didn't have to hear what I've heard before. I decided to go with *"Natural Mystic"* by *Bob Marley & The Wailers*. I fell onto my bed trying to relax reflecting on my hand I gave away to Tone, and even though my plan for the night was to end my drought, I'm happy that I was able to keep my promise.

I could feel my eyelids get heavy, and before I turned my desk lamp off, I'd hear a slight knock on my door. *What the fuck!* I thought. I leaped out of bed and checked my drawer for condoms; maybe Tone pussy'ed out, and my original plan to end my drought was about to commence. I rushed to the door, breathed into my palm to check if I had hot breath, thankfully I was good. I slowly opened the door, and before I could open the door fully Tone bulls through.

"What's up?" Tone asked.

"What the fuck? What are you doing?" I asked confused.

"Dude, I don't know how to ask her." Tone said.

"Ask her what?" I asked.

"You know, to um come to my room so I could fuck the shit out of her." Tone said.

"First of all, if you say those exact words, I'm sure she wouldn't do shit with you," I said.

I opened my door slightly to check on Julie, and she was laying on the couch covered completely.

"I don't know man, just be smooth. Go up to her, and whisper, 'Let's go to my bedroom,' and softly hold her hand and lead her to your room." I said.

"That's not bad." Tone said.

"Dude, what's the worst that could happen?" I asked.

"She could shut me down, and I'd be forced to take the "walk of shame." Tone said while pacing in my bedroom.

"You heard her earlier when she said that she loves it when a man asks. She's not going to ask, so you might as well just take your shot brother." I said.

I grabbed Tone by the shoulders and told him "Snap out of it, and show Julie what's up?"

"Okay, fuck it! I'm doing it." Tone said motivated ready for battle.

Tone walked out my door swiftly; I, on the other hand, peaked from the edge of my door like I was some kind of pervert curious to see if my promise was going to transpire—I had never been so excited for Tone. He leaned over Julie and whispers to her. From my view, all I could see was the back of Julie's head. Then Tone reaches for her hand,

and I see Julie's head nod "no." I instantly turned away not wanting to see Tones reaction of being shut down certainly never wanting to see his "walk of shame." I dig my head into my palm crushed over Tones defeat when Tone walked back into my bedroom somewhat slamming my door understandably.

"Dude, I'm so sorry man," I said.

"It's all good; maybe it's for the best. Besides, she's here for you dawg." Tone said.

"What? Maybe originally, but by the end of our poker night, she was all over you." I said.

"I know, I think I took too long to make a move, and maybe she thought I was a pussy or something." Tone said.

"Well, I have to be honest I'm exhausted. I'm sure if Brandy never left than Julie would without a doubt be in here rather than out there, and you'd surely be tossing Brandy." I said.

"Go ahead man, don't worry about me. I'm not pissed or anything." Tone said.

"Are you sure?" I said.

Tone puts his hand on my shoulder when suddenly my stomach growls loud enough to wake Julie an entire room and hall way away.

"Dang, are you hungry?" Tone asked.

"Always my man, always," I said.

"Shit! Now you're making me hungry."

"To be honest, I much rather eat a JIB than risk Julie turning me down," I said.

"Really? I thought you were determined to end your drought?" Tone asked.

"Yeah, but I may need the strength," I said realizing I was about to cross a line I never thought I would pass.

I peeked out the door to check on Julie, and she was sleeping on the couch appearing ready for me to make a move.

"Listen, why don't we go to JIB-U, and bring something back for Julie in case she asks." Tone said.

"Come on, how stupid would it be if we left a hot chic for a fucking burger and breakfast sandwich?" I asked.

"Why don't we wait a while until we know Julie is deeply asleep, then we can sneak out of here like nothing happened." Tone asked.

A deep silence overcast my bedroom as Tone and I knew we were about to embark on something unprecedented. A small part of me believed Tone was trying to sabotage my task for the night, but the idea of slapping my taste buds with a double bacon cheeseburger was flooding any desire to end my drought.

"O—kay."

Tone and I waited in my room for another 30 minutes talking about whether we were going to get a burger or a breakfast sandwich, and who would win in a fight between Ronald McDonald or Jack. I wasn't sure if our conversation was more stupid than the fact that I was going to pass up ending my drought for a big, fat juicy burger. Predictably, Tone and I would sneak out of our apartment to pick up some *Jack-In-The-Box* and sneak back in as if we were burglars to our own place and watch a pirated movie all while Julie slept ALONE on our couch that night.

Eventually, Tone and Francis would get back together all while my drought continued. The following morning I'd check to see if Julie was gone, and indeed she was along with the idea of the T-N-T Experience.

> *"Yes! Can **WE** order two double bacon cheeseburger combos with sourdough buns and curly fries?" I asked the drive-thru attendant.*

*"Yes, is there anything else?" The drive-thru attendant asked.*

*"Can you also throw in two double-sausage breakfast sand-*
*wiches with both drinks large Cokes?"*

*"No problem, will that be all?"*

*"And two chocolate desserts please, that's it."*

*"Okay, drive up, and I'll give you your total."*

# THE DAY SUPERMAN DIED

$\mathcal{M}$Y FATHER GREW UP in a town called Gregory, Texas during the 50s and 60s. Gregory is a neighboring town of Corpus Christi with a population of about 3,000 residents. During my father's childhood, he and his family lived a humble life, a migrant life. They traveled in season to California, Washington, and Michigan to work the fields. When they would come back home to Gregory, his parents and grandparents picked cotton in the surrounding rural towns. My father always told me stories how his family worked from 5:30 in the morning until 8 p.m. every day hunched over under the blazing sun just to get paid $1.50 per 100-pounds they picked in those 10-12-foot cotton satchels. My father as a 10-year-old boy set a goal every day to pick 500- pounds so he would at least make $7.50 and give five of those dollars to his family all while keeping $2.50; which eventually went towards his family anyways.

When my dad graduated high school, he used everything he saved from working the fields and bought my grandparents a car just to make life a little easier. I always felt whenever he'd tell me that story that in a strange way my father bought them that car so his parents (my grand-parents) could experience what "new" was, and simply smile. But that has always been the person my dad is, someone who sacrifices just to see the people around him smile; even if it's just for a moment.

Eventually, he met my mom who also grew up working in the fields.

During the 50s and 60s, it was common for Mexican American families to migrate during the school year. Considering both my parents were migrants we came from a family that is 5th or 6th generation American; even before the Mexican American war.

Directly after high school, my father moved away from Gregory to the Rio Grande Valley; McAllen to be specific which was a two-and-a-half-hour drive south. He worked his way from sweeping a broom to a store manager, to eventually owner of a nuts and bolts distributor. My father's work ethic was unparalleled to anything I've ever seen. His hands, although it had been decades since he worked in the fields, were marked with calluses in groves resembling the crop-fields he used to work. Growing up, I never heard him, or my mom complain about work. They always approached their job with a smile and the necessary tenacity to be great. Although I'm sure they had plenty of days they wanted to call in, they simply did their job to provide. Their example is everything to me and is to this day contagious. I've always believed that if I had 10% of their traits then I can achieve anything I set my mind to.

When my father moved down to the Rio Grande Valley, he joined many organizations, but because he had never been the type to stand in the background and just listen, he always put himself in the front lines and helped all that he could. My father became an "idea man" and a leader in the business community contributing towards the growth of McAllen, which eventually would become one of the fastest growing cities in America.

My father learned how cutthroat business was and how necessary an education was needed to succeed. Considering Dad came from a high school where racism was rampant; and grew up thinking that Mexicans were not allowed to go to college, as my father and the other minorities in his school were instead taught trades such as being a plumber or an electrician— the concept of college was never an option which was expressed by his teachers.

After years of marriage, and when my older sister and I were nine and five respectively, both my parents decided that they had to both go to college so that they could not only provide for my family but be the examples for my sister and me and eventually my younger brother. Both my parents decided to go back to school at the same time. Besides working full-time, they both went to school full-time. I recall my sister and I often waiting outside their classroom at the university after they finished a long day of work. Imagine today's parents leaving their children out of sight. Jesus how times have changed.

Both my parents graduated, my father a year before my mother from Pan American University. I recall my father's graduation party, and even though I was eight years old seeing my dad in his funny all-black cap and gown filled me with a sense of pride that infiltrated through my body for the first time in my life. It was a feeling that I had never felt before, but I knew that it was a special feeling that I could only pray I returned to him one day. The following year I regained that sense of pride during Mom's graduation.

Seeing my parents walk across the stage to accept their diploma meant everything to me because I saw a dream realized by both my parents who were told their entire lives that they were never meant to go to college much less dream, even if they were wearing that funny all-black cap and gown.

My mom became an elementary teacher for 25 years, while my father taught mathematics in high school and college, but eventually dove into financing by the time I entered high school for the next 15 years.

***

I was 24 years old and convinced that college just wasn't for me; talk about being the opposite of who my father and mother were. I joined the workforce, and considering I had aspirations of becoming the next great screenwriter, the furthest I ever went into the film industry was working on a film as a P.A. in the Austin/New Braunfels area. During this time in my life, I was such a dreamer. It wasn't so much that I didn't want to go to college, it was more because I wanted to be in the movie business so bad, I figured hands-on experience in the film industry had to be better than going to school for filmmaking.

After completing the film as a P.A. in the Austin/ New Braunfels area in 2005, I came home with aspirations to continue working on my dream of becoming a screenwriter. With the great connections I made from working on that film, I sincerely thought I was on the verge of breaking through and having my dreams come true.

One day, my father and I went for a walk. On this walk, he asked me.

"Son, I want you to come work with me as a loan processor. It pays well, we're very busy, and I need a helping hand."

For me, I wanted to work on my next story, but I saw that my dad needed me, and I figured "how great would it be to work with my father." Also, I'd be out of work by 5 p.m. so I'd have plenty of time to work on my craft. I gladly accepted, and within a few weeks, I was completely hooked working as a loan processor at *Finance Capital.*

Meeting customers, working on files, and learning a new language of sorts was stimulating my mind. The natural high I received when closing a loan was unreal, and I was sincerely having a great time working. All these new aspects of learning I was gaining just by being a loan processor helped me grow as a person. I honestly felt that I was contributing to helping families accomplish their dreams of owning a home. For the first time in my life, I felt like an asset in the workforce. Besides learning a new language and closing loans my favorite time of day was lunch. Not because it was time off, but because I'd got to spend every day with my dad figuring out ways to solve the entire world's problems, which I must say we both came up with some great ideas. Everything from President Bush's dumbass policies, to the Chicano movement— it was a glorious time in my life. I loved every second I was there with my dad.

Then came September of 2007 when the economy crashed especially in housing. We were already feeling the decline in processed home loans as restrictions were getting tighter by the day. When that FATAL September happened, it felt like it was pointed directly at us *Finance Capital*. Within the same day, it was as if the table was taken from right underneath us. When I first arrived at *Finance Capital*, we were closing 25 plus loans a month to eventually one if we were lucky. Ultimately, my father and my beloved lunches came to a screeching halt, and for the first time, I ate alone in frustration concerned for my dad.

Dad's employees trickled down and down until it was eventually just him and me. The luminous man that my dad had always been and that I've always known began to wilt. Thankfully because of his unmatched optimism, all the chinks in his armor that he endured that year was polished clean as he worked just as hard as he ever did. That work ethic and attitude must've stemmed from his days as a ten-year-old picking those 500-pounds of cotton. Now, some forty-six years later as if time stood still his work ethic was put to the test just to keep the lights on at *Finance Capital*— I loved our odds.

As much as I enjoyed my job as a loan processor and working with my dad, I did take advantage of my father when I worked with him. I'd often come in an hour late and left an hour early. In retrospect, I often believe that if I took my job seriously, maybe *Finance Capital* would still be open for business. Eventually, the market crashed claiming my father's business of 15 years. No matter how broad and strong my dad's shoulders were when August of 2008 came around, that's when I would see Superman die.

***

The month leading to that fateful day in August 2008 my admiration for my father had never been brighter. I knew my father was feeling all these pressures especially when we were about to close a loan. With the market changing, many new restrictions were implemented whether it was opening or closing a loan. Often when we were in the final step(s) to close an account, during the 11th hour, we'd predictably, receive a phone call from the banker explaining why the bank or buyer had to pull-out from the loan completely as if it was on purpose. Suddenly my love for the job turned to hate when I'd be forced to break the bad news to my dad that the loan we worked so hard on fell through at the last *moment*. I could tell my father wanted to explode in complete frustration, but nope, he always understood that it was business, and would simply put the file away all while putting his straight face on for my sake, and for that, I could never be more grateful.

I've learned from my father that all that ever mattered to him was his love for his family and God. He never complained about anything no matter how difficult life would get and believe me we had plenty of trials and tribulations through the years. I just wish I could have given him the reprieve he deserved while I grew up. Imagine all the bull-shit I compiled upon everything else Dad was enduring whether it was my hi-jinx in high school, getting arrested (multiple times,) or asking for money to pay off my debts.

For my father, his way of thinking when life got tough was "It could always be worse." Now I understand that quote may apply to some, but for me, it truly got me through rough times I thought I'd never survive, especially now as an obese man.

I must admit it was life draining to see my father's dream of being an entrepreneur fall apart in front of my eyes. From the days of picking cotton as a little boy, to now shutting the doors to *Finance Capital* all while keeping a smile on his face, makes me crave for 10% of the man he is.

***

One late August night, my father and I were working on an account trying to figure out how to close a loan. Before the housing market collapsed, this particular loan would have been elementary to close, but because of the newly found chaotic economic downturn, banks implemented many restrictions and red-tape making what was once a "routine" home loan now become nearly impossible to close. I vividly recall working through the night trying to solve this account. Although we had other loans to work on, this specific one was the closest to closing, and needed as much focus so we could put this file in the book and label it "closed," which to be honest had been weeks if not months since we had finalized a single loan. We both knew the odds of closing this loan was slim to none; we worked diligently certainly desperately trying to find a way to beat through the banks "new" unreachable requirements like a once proud boxing champ getting pummeled, and throwing lethargic haymakers wishing one punch will land— nothing was connecting. We were at the mercy of the banker waiting for their call to inform us that everything was "good to go," and the loan had been approved to close. Except, when we finally received the call there was no good news, and we were forced to take the loss, and simply put the file away in defeat.

On this specific night, I knew it was over. I couldn't look my dad in the eyes, because I knew throughout his optimism there would be disappointment causing me to lose it completely and probably weep in frustration. Unfortunately, seeing my dad during this chaotic time put on a "front" for my sake had become all too customary. Before, whenever I'd give him the "bad news" that any loan was not going to close; Dad would simply sigh and move onto the next loan while whistling Dixie.

I'll be honest, on this particular night seeing my dad put the file away with a strange smile on his face only screamed fraudulence to me as I knew he was disappointed. Even the way he filed the loan as if he was letting go of a lost love screamed that he knew that the *Finance Capital* days were numbered. Seeing my dad linger to the edge of the manila folder hoping for some kind of miracle, made me want to put my arm around him and tell him, "everything is going to be okay" like in the movies, but I just sat there. I just sat there looking at Dad in the distance take a harpoon to the heart as we were both unclear about what tomorrow would behold. For the first time in my life, I needed my dad to tell me "everything is going to be okay."

***

I was then typing in a "new" hopeful account. My office shared a wall with my father, and while I was almost near completion of the application ready to fax away every page to our banker, I heard someone enter our building. Normally, I would greet the person, and direct them to my father's office for a consultation, but I instantly became rattled as the unknown customer's boots stomped and echoed through the hallway startling me— something was up. The rustling of his keys echoed through our building sending shivers down my spine stopping me in my tracks as if I was stuck in a force field of sorts.

Since Dad's office was closest to the entrance, perhaps he could greet this "disturbance," instead I heard this man barge into my father's office, and with a stern bombastic hick-like voice asked.

"Are you the owner of *Finance Capital LLC*? Emphasizing *"LLC"* like it was alien to him.

From the neighboring room, I clenched my fist as my body had become flushed with goose-bumps and I didn't know why. His deep daunting voice resembled a cowboy drawl capable of making John Wayne shake in his boots.

"Yes sir, how can I help you?" My dad said.

"You need to clean out your stuff and be out of this building by Saturday night."

"No problem." My father said as if he was expecting such a request.

My fist clenched even tighter as my middle knuckle resembled the Rock of Gibraltar. Although I was ready to burst through the wall like the Hulk and smash that hick for speaking to my dad like he did, I just stood there paralyzed with fear and simply couldn't move. My eyes began to water, and my knees rattled like a withering old man as my thoughts were flooded with red. All I wanted at that exact moment was to see who this piece of shit was, but I was stuck in his forcefield.

I heard him turn in what sounded like an about-face, as his boots and keys rustled out of our building. As soon as the man exited, my body went back to normal. At that instant, I wanted to go out the door, and chase down the cocksucka who had the balls to tell the greatest man who ever lived what to do as if he was some judge passing down a life sentence. Out of frustration, I threw haymakers into the air as the cutting wind from my then cut arms broke the silence.

It was eerily quiet throughout my office for the next 10 minutes. Out of respect for my father, instead of inquiring what the ruckus was all about, I gave him his own time to register what just happened as if I had the right.

While I paced back and forth in my office waiting for my tears to dry, I couldn't get that piece of shit's voice out of my head. "YOU NEED TO CLEAN OUT YOUR STUFF AND BE OUT OF THIS BUILDING BY SATURDAY NIGHT!" Kept rumbling in my head amplifying and amplifying with every step I took. In my 27 years I been alive, I had never heard anyone talk to my father like that, and I wasn't sure how to process it. I just wish I wasn't there to have heard it in the first place.

After I cooled down, I walked out of my office and into my father's, and of course, he was hard at work as if nothing ever occurred. With every step I took into his office, I felt like I was seeing my father for the first time in this new "dim" light. *Why wasn't he pissed? Why didn't he go after that man, and beat the fuck out of him? I certainly would have tag-teamed with my father and curbed him.* As my dad's nose was burrowed into a file, I didn't see the Superman that he always was anymore. Now, the man who had the respect of everyone was gone. The man who was never defeated was now crushed by the "disturbance" that walked in that day. I wanted then to grab my father by the collar and shout some sense into him, so I could see some real emotion especially after some *Man, Being,* or *Doomsday* himself had just walked in like he owned the place, and simply told my dad that his dream was over. After I was done gawking at my father for what seemed an eternity, as it was just a mere second, I decided not to bring up the "disturbance" or in this case "Superman's Doomsday." Instead, my father discussed the file, and what needed to be done tomorrow as if nothing happened. Considering the instant changes in emotion, I was enduring just being in his office; I was thankful for the familiarity.

***

By this time, I was gaining my weight back. When I first started working with my father, I came in weighing 282-pounds and would lose a 105-pounds in about four months. My father always told the story how he came in one day with pan dulce (Mexican sweetbread,) and while everyone took a piece according to their personality, I would simply grab the bag and sniff the alluring scent of my heritage and begrudgingly put it away. That's how focused I was on those four months of losing weight. Of course, this was the era when I lived with Olivia (a family friend), and eventually with Tone. I'm not sure if it was the stock market crash combined with seeing my father get bombarded with the times, but it was during those last few months where I'd begun to gain my weight back. By the time we closed the doors that Saturday night after the "disturbance or Doomsday" told my father to get the "fuck out," I weighed a solid 256-pounds.

That Saturday finally came, and of course, I helped my father move out of his office. Although I saw a new confusing version of my father, he was still the same guy. Strange enough, we had a great time moving out and closing *Finance Capital*. My father talked about the plans he had for his business and told me that he could no longer pay me, and if I wanted to move back home, I was more than welcome. At the time I had plenty of savings to stay out on my own for a few more months, and find work elsewhere, but I wanted to move home to be with my father and family, as I felt in a selfish way my presence was essential, and maybe being together would make this transition go smoother.

That night I gave my dad a rare deep hug and assured him that everything was going to be okay— at that moment I felt I was earning that 10% I've always craved. Years later, I often reflect on that fateful August day. I had always labeled it the day "Superman died," because that was the first time in my life I heard my father have no answer.

In the comic series when Superman dies, he eventually resurrects even stronger and focuses on becoming a greater version than he ever was. As for my dad, he rebounded becoming stronger and more focused than ever. It was in this transition where he'd become the GREATEST version of himself— Superman.

# THE BOTTOM OF THE BARREL

THE DAY AFTER I helped my dad move out of his building, my life and style fundamentally shifted in a 24-hour span. Sure, I may have had a week to figure something(s) out, but in all honesty, I wanted to be with my dad, and do anything I could to recoup his cape.

That Saturday night, I remembered buying a large combo meal, which by this time I was well into my second bound of gaining weight. The following morning, I had told Tone about my dad's situation; thankfully he understood that I would be going through a rather drastic life change. So with my tail between my legs, and at my local bar I decided after my third shot of Tequila that I would follow through, and move back home at the ripe old age of 27.

I recalled thinking *I'm 27 years old gaining ALL my weight back, unemployed, and living at home.* No matter how optimistic I was when I committed to my father after that long day of moving, it suddenly felt like a death trap. Growing up a major *Seinfeld* fan it became clear that I was becoming George Costanza or in this case "Jorge Costanzo," the Mexican version.

Within the buzz of my third Tequila shot going on four, I knew I had to find a silver lining, something that I needed at this exact second as I downed my fourth shot so that I could claim some kind of victory especially after the long hard emotional week I had just endured. After

I opened my eyes from the aftertaste of the Tequila, I looked around the bar hoping that I appeared invisible to my fellow "daylight barflies" when suddenly, I saw a cute girl sitting at the far left of the bar shuffling through textbooks like a madman or in this case a madwoman. Instead of crushing on her because she was damn cute, I envied her. Not because she was studying at a bar while also fighting her demons, but at least she had a focus, and by the way she was darting through that textbook the size of the 9/11 *Commission Report*, I would've killed to switch places with her.

I knew I was driving home or to my mom and dad's place, so I asked the bartender for a glass of water to sober up, and that's when it hit me suddenly: *I should go back to school except this time give my maximum effort.* As much as it pained me to admit it, I'd collect unemployment that my dad offered, so I could get a head start on my education and use the time off to focus on my studies because I was never the greatest of students. So, within those few weeks, I was unemployed, living at home at the age of 27 hurdling towards a 2XL t-shirt, but at least I was registered for school. Being at the bottom of the barrel, it seemed as if the lid was loosened and I was provided with some life.

***

Sadly, this endeavor lasted until I was 34 years old. Of course, I would go back to work but never earn enough to live on my own. When I kept trying to climb out of the barrel, there always seemed to be something holding me back. Between the closing *of Finance Capital* and going back to school that following year I would weigh in at a full rounded 301-pounds. After completing my first year of college, I became motivated to lose weight again -*because of the college girls*- and would drop 70-pounds, weighing in at 231-pounds by my second year of community college. Unfortunately, it seemed that day I weighed in and saw the scale read

231- pounds, it was like a red alarm expressing that I did a "great job," and now have a burger, and a burger I did. As a matter of fact, I did so many burgers that by the time I graduated in 2014 almost 6 years after enrolling in community college, I weighed a shocking 401-pounds.

That last semester when I breached the 401-pound barrier, walking from class to class had become extremely taxing on my body even to the point where I considered it a sport. Bobbing and weaving through the student body on the way to class as a 401-pound monster was physically and emotionally exhausting.

That final year, I also began looking for a new job; a career of sorts whether it be in teaching or coaching. I figured I'd get a head start on my profession before I graduated, but the only problem was that no one was hiring, even though every one of those jobs I applied for had a "help wanted" sign outside their establishment.

Now as a large man you understand when your weight becomes a spectacle of sorts, and your mind defaults to thinking that your weight becomes a crucial factor in the hiring process. Now whether that's fair or not, I would never say because our Earth is as superficial as it has ever been, myself included. Imagine if I were alive during the Roman Empire era where large men were classified as rich than I would've been Julius Caesar (except without the back-stabbing.) Unfortunately, that was not the case, and in reality, having to endure this hindrance of judgment because of my size is a reality that I had to deal with, and a challenge I gladly accepted. I recalled walking into those establishments that were looking for work, and when I asked for an application I would always, and I mean always get this quick scan from the secretary like those girls from *Luka Bar*, except this time the scans were of disgust and disbelief. I could still see in their eyes as if they were witnessing history seeing someone as big as me, I could only imagine their thoughts such as, "I've never seen a belly that big!" or "how can a man grow breasts that big?" It was humiliating, to say the least; even more so as I type this very sentence. Looking back, I probably could never work at most of those establishments anyways because of the physical requirements they required. Besides, whenever I turned in a completed application and talked to the manager not only would I get scanned, I knew he or she would have never hired me because of the "liability" issue which was valid, but I expected.

\*\*\*

The other aspect of being at the bottom of the barrel was simply living at home. In this duration of my life, my youngest brother of 10 years had moved out and was living the life I used to live in all variations. I saw him having a blast with his buddies and jumping from girl to girl until he found his mate. All while I spent my weekends stuffing my face and regretting what I was missing out on but never garnered the strength to lose the weight or find a *Jeep*. So, between the ages of 28-34 with about 50% of that time also being unemployed, it wasn't that hard to believe that I'd made it to an eventual 401-pounds.

Now, one wondered how I obtained the money to buy all those meals which usually came at the cost of $10-$15 a trip, multiplied by three to four times a day. So, how did I compile $40-$60 a day unemployed? Well, those times I wasn't working, I collected unemployment, and those 400 dollars I received every two weeks, I used to hit those fast food joints. When money was tight, unfortunately, I had no girl, or bills because I lived with Mom and Dad. Thus, after getting my unemployment check that first week, I would spend the majority of the money on high-end fast food joints. When that second week came, and I would have $50 to a $100 left to my name, that's when I would fully exploit, and I mean exploit the dollar menu to the fullest, which made it possible to attack with extreme force.

The "cherry on top" of being at the bottom of the barrel was missing out of my brother Jesse's ascension towards adulthood. Until then I missed out on his youth because I attributed him as ten years younger than me. So, when he was 5,6,7, or 8 years old, instead of being the cool older brother, I was an absolute cocksucka only consumed in myself to ever give a fuck about how much he needed that "older brother" influence all while I was immersed in my high school years. As my brother hit the ages of 18 to 24, I predictably wasn't there for him again. While he transitioned to adulthood, here I was transitioning from a 2XL to a whopping 6XL all while in a reclusive state of self-absorption. I'm not talking about the psychological term; I mean self-absorption as in absorbing everything in sight– in its literal gluttonous form. Just writing about my brother and I's relationship breaks my heart, because it was something I could cure by simply just being with him and creating more moments from the very few we had. I am proud however over the recent years that our relationship began to build, and along with a number 2 from *Whataburger* my relationship with my brother was really the only thing I'd ever craved.

> "Can **WE** order four double cheeseburgers from your dollar menu?" I asked.
> "Yes, you can, would you like to add a dollar fries and a dollar Coke to your order?"
> "…yes, can you make it three orders of dollar fries, and make the Coke a large please?"
> "No problem, will that be all?" The drive-thru attendant asked.

*"Yes, can you add a dollar fried chicken burger please?"*
*I asked.*
*"No problem."*

# II

# THE LIFE
*of a junky*

# THE FALL: VOL. II

*W*HEN I WENT FROM 282-pounds to 179-pounds the first time I ever dieted, I got there in about four months of eating nothing but low carb meals and running. I started with forcing myself to run a ½ mile and walking the rest completing one mile a day. Eventually, that mile turned to two miles to eventually three complete miles. Then I transitioned to running. Along with running a mile non-stop, I eventually increased to 5 miles and by the time I reached a 179-pounds I was running 8-12 miles at a sensational pace.

I, of course, lost my way, and in no time in about a two-year span would jump from 179- pounds to 301-pounds exactly. I'm not sure how I got to 301; all I know is that I went through a tough time from my dad having to close his business, to moving back home being unemployed to gaining my bad habits of eating uncontrollably again. During this time in my life, I endured an emotional and physical strain that I had never felt before in all honesty. I guess as cliché as it may sound "I was eating my emotions."

I'd begin to lose weight when my older sister Karina challenge me to a weekly weigh in diet. For my sister, she was beginning to feel self-conscious after giving birth to my amazing nephew Zeke who just turned two years old, and my sister was struggling with her weight. We agreed to a challenge and helped one another, and within a three-month span, I lost

70-pounds reaching 231-pounds and felt motivated after my first year of college. As for my sister, she didn't have the success I did, but she certainly lost weight to the point where she regained confidence again, becoming the strong sister I've always known. Of course, similar to when I weighed 282- pounds, and 301-pounds, I can't pinpoint an exact *moment* from when I lost my way, but I would account it to self-ignorance, believing I could eat any meal I want and not gain a single ounce. So, instead of learning my lesson from my second voyage on the way to 301, I fell off the wagon, except I wouldn't just fall off the wagon, but I'd fall off, and fledge onto a deep vortex the size of two proverbial Mount Everest and eventually weigh 401-pounds.

To be a part of the 300-pound club is one thing and is something you often see whether it be professional football players or an account of someone losing their way physically which in this day and age is quite common. There are usually two ways that someone can go when they hit the 300-pound club: they can lose pounds and get to their ideal weight which is a common and able feat that many people can relate to. The other way is to lose yourself completely and reach realms where breaking the 400, 500, or 600-pound plus barriers occur and you're in the truest of words... fucked.

For me when I hit the 400-pound threshold (401) to be exact, it became exactly what it was– a threshold. It became two Everest's. Each Everest would be losing a hundred pounds each and eventually weighing under 200. Just thinking of it was mentally exhausting. I'm not sure how I got to 401-pounds from 231-pounds, but it felt like it happened even quicker from when I went from 179-pounds to 301-pounds a few years earlier.

Life changes when you hit the 300 to 400-pound barriers. Although they are a hundred pounds apart, they're different in the greatest of forms.

As silly as it sounds, wanting to lose 100 pounds from 300 is an "Everest" within itself, but it is doable. But when someone hits the 400 plus barrier, it becomes a mental fuck that unless you have weighed anywhere near 400 pounds, or fuck it 330 pounds, you simply begin to understand the challenges you have whether they are physically, mentally, and probably most importantly emotionally for which all three go hand in hand.

For anyone who gets to either the 300 or 400-pound breaking point, we understand that this is all self-inflicting. We don't expect any sympathy or empathy from anyone because we know and pray that it's temporary, and just like anything else we know that it's all going to come back to what we need to do to get into a healthy state, or as I like to measure it as "a decent size t-shirt." What we want more than anything is for people to understand that we don't look at you as being "lucky" that you don't share our addiction; but understand that we know that we are in a state of constant surveillance. We know that when we go out to eat, that people are expecting us to eat a salad. We know that when we go out, that people are expecting us to dress to size. We know that when we go out, you'll stare. We know that when we go out, we must not express that we are happy with our size. Most importantly, we just want everyone to know that your concern for us is valid, and taken, but understand what we're enduring every day for the majority of us is a non-stop constant mind fuck of weight-loss or anything that has to do with health. From waking up until our eyes close at night the constant thought of our weight saturates our every thought process— no pun intended.

> "Can **WE** order three breakfast tacos, two of which are
> chorizo and egg, and the other a bacon, potato, egg, and
> cheese taco with a large soda?" I asked.
> "Just to inform you, sir, our medium is a 32 ounce, and

*our large is a 64 ounce. Is that okay? The drive-through attendant asked.*

*"Sure, in that case, can you make it a grape soda?"*

*"Okay, is there anything else?"*

*I perused the menu and noticed they also sold doughnuts.*

*"Can WE also have a ½ dozen of your glazed doughnuts with chocolate milk?"*

*"No problem, will that be all?"*

*"…Um… let me have–; never mind, that'll be all," I said.*

# HUMBLE PIE: VOL. I

$\mathscr{G}$ROWING UP, I NEVER enjoyed school. I would love to say that I was an "A" student, received a full-ride academic scholarship to the University of Texas or my dream school Georgetown University, but unfortunately, I was stuck in a rotation of remedial courses. In Texas, for every season there is either a seasonal state test administered, or some bull-shit benchmark, and if you didn't do too hot you were placed in these remedial courses where basics were skipped, and creativity was left to perish. Those classes became more of a social club than a high-level institute, leaving me to graduate in the bottom 10% of my class.

After I graduated high school, I spent the next ten years flunking in and out of college to the point where I was content with the idea that "school was simply not for me." Well, as I stated previously, I thoroughly enjoyed being a loan processor with aspirations of becoming a real estate mogul. That was until that fateful day I heard that man with his thundering boots, and what I always thought how God would sound like tell my dad: "BE OUT BY SATURDAY." Like a jolt of lightning, I decided my only way out of being in the "bottom of the barrel" was simply going back to school and finding something I'd love to do for the rest of my life, but most importantly protect myself from financial suffrage.

After two years of junior college, I finally transferred to my local university, the University of Texas-Pan American like both my parents and eventually my older sister. I pursued a degree in Kinesiology (iron-ically), and a minor in history. By the time I graduated, I had switched degree plans and graduated with a degree in history (Arts & Humanities.)

My first day as a transfer to Pan American was a 7 a.m. course in swimming. Now, I didn't sign up for this class because let's face it the last thing I wanted to do was see the water rise an inch or two all because I entered it. When I signed up for this class it was part of an activities course that had no detail of which sports I was going to learn; it was just titled *Sports Athletics*. I naturally assumed that it would be a football or basketball class which would've been amazing since I was a pretty good street quarterback back in my 32-inch waist days, and of course basketball in which I was better of the two.

Normally, when the first day of class commences, it's usually an "introductory" day entailing who the instructor is, classroom expectations and details of the syllabus, in all concluding in about 20 minutes. Instead, about a minute after class should've begun, the teacher walked in, and of course, she was stunning. I was 30 at the time I transferred to the university, and she looked my age. Predictably, my first thoughts were if *I was in shape, I could totally pick her up, and earn an "A" by commencing in that old cliché of a student/professor relationship.*

After the hot professor stepped into the classroom, I instantly noticed her vibrant smile. Her smile was so radiant that it distracted me from my impending embarrassing death, and it was in her hand. As she squeezed through me and the apparent aisle that I consumed, I noticed that she was carrying a weighing scale. *WHAT THE FUCK!* I thought. I looked at the other students to see if they noticed or had the same concern I did. *Why the fuck does she have a scale on her?* I thought. My heart beat dropped to about a thump a second, as I burst into a cold sweat as numerous thoughts swirled through my mind.

"Everyone up and get into a straight line." She commanded.

She didn't even introduce herself or review the syllabus. *What kind of bull-shit instructor is this?* As we stood in line, she explained why she had the scale and an apparent measuring tape, but I couldn't hear a fucking thing, as I was trying to figure out a way to get out of this potentially devastating trap and avoid this weigh-in.

Everyone including the cute girls got in line. I tried my best to procrastinate, when I deceptively packed my backpack, with the intentions of squirming out of class, and take the zero for the day, which I was happy to sacrifice instead of being humiliated once I stepped onto that scale. After I put my book and notebook into my bag, I stood and tried my best to exit when the instructor said.

"No one leaves until everyone weighs-in, so we can discuss the syllabus." I put my bag down and looked up at the ceiling in defeat. By this time, my face was blue, and I would purposely be the last one in line. My thinking was, *Hopefully, by the time I weigh myself a few of the students especially the cute girls would leave class and miss what would be a great conversation piece during their lunch break.*

To my surprise, the line took longer than expected. I prayed that we'd run out of time before it was my turn to step on to the scale. It was ten minutes until class let out when the instructor said.

"Since we are close to running out of time, we are going to forget the measuring tape, and just weigh in."

*FUCK ME!* I thought.

*Why couldn't it be the other way around? I'd proudly have my waist measured over a weigh-in any day of the week. Just being on display on a scale I'm not so sure could even support me, was by far more humiliating.* I thought. The line started zooming, and what was originally being whispered about each student's waistline between teacher and student was now being shouted across the classroom for everyone to hear. The sounds of 149, 155, 183, 201, 101 pounds grabbed my attention. I tried remembering the last time I weighed myself and recalled that it was back to when I weighed 301-pounds, just after I had lost 70-pounds over a year and a half earlier, only to gain every pound back. *Did I weigh myself 4 months ago? Or was it 3 months ago?* I couldn't remember. All I knew was that my eating habits had gotten worse since I last weighed-in, and for the first time in my life I'd know, and in front of an audience of complete strangers soon to be friends and study buddies, I was about to cross over the 300-pound threshold for the first time in public– a ring of sweat would darken my collar.

"And your name?" The instructor asked the student in front of me.

"Adrian Velasco."

"Okay, Adrian please step on the scale."

I watched as Adrian approached the scale. Besides the small talk, he and I engaged in from standing in this line about my Dallas Cowboys, and his love for the New England Patriots. I couldn't help but envy him; I wanted to be him. I mean he couldn't weigh more than a 145-pounds soaking wet. Even though he was no taller than 5'6, I'd definitely just for this weigh-in do anything to be in his shoes.

"One hundred- and forty-three-pounds Adrian," the instructor said.

I noticed Adrian nod in disappointment, as he turned and whispered to me.

"Dude, when I graduated high school, I weighed a 140-pounds solid steel; I need to diet." I fauxly smiled, and wanted to beat the fuck out of him, and tell him "shut the fuck up brah; one of my chins weighs more than you." It was my turn.

"Your name?" The instructor asked.

I looked at her straight in the eyes as my heart raced faster than any student would in the swimming pool that semester. She had to know how uncomfortable I was feeling, right?

"Um… Tre, Tre Garcia?"

"Please stand on the scale," she said with no remorse.

*FUCKING BITCH!* I thought.

All the conversation in the classroom stopped. I knew if I looked back at the class then I'd get those swift rubbernecks appearing like my weigh-in was no big deal or some kind of courtesy that I was not a spectacle of sorts, which was by far more insulting. I took a deep breath and approached the scale. With each step echoing off the silent brick walled classroom, I stepped onto the scale and looked up to the ceiling defeated, humiliated, and certainly destroyed beyond recognition. I closed my eyes and exhaled.

After what seemed like an eternity as I was sure the scale had never endured such a mountain of a man standing on top of it, the hot instructor said nonchalantly: "320-pounds." She wrote in her clipboard somewhat disappointed. I turned to my new fellow classmates. Half the students had their mouths completely agape, as their jaws had fallen to the core of the Earth, while the other half turned their head away on a swivel. I walked to my desk trying to appear as if I didn't give a fuck, and literally squeezed into my desk. I sat next to Adrian who in the short period had already befriended me only to state:

"Dude, you weigh the same as Leonard Davis," Adrian said.

Leonard Davis at one time was the starting guard for the Dallas Cowboys and an ex-Texas Longhorn I might add. Adrian's comment truly made me laugh, as I saw in his eyes no judgment, just a guy trying to make me laugh, and he succeeded. Most would've found it insulting, but like most large people, we know cruel intent when we see or hear it, and Adrian was just being a clown, and actually salvaged the class for me throughout the semester, as we would become great friends only confirming that he never had any ill-will towards me– Thank you, Adrian.

> *"Can **WE** have an order of four carne guisada tacos, an enchilada plate, and a large soda with a tres leches cake please?" I asked the drive-thru attendant.*
> *"Yes, anything else?"*
> *A bowl of menudo would be bad-ass to add, but that weigh-in today messed me up. I thought.*
> *"That'll be all."*

# SECOND OF THE MONTH

$\mathcal{M}$ONTHS AFTER THE JULIE debacle, Tone and I were on a fast track of gaining more weight. Our nights and weekends would consist of a large pizza pie *-one for each-* and watching pirated movies until sun-up. Occasionally, we'd go out to our local bar named *Tio Chuy's* and drink ourselves to a late-night smorgasbord of *Whataburger* breakfast sandwiches, only to conclude with us both crashed out on our sofa like two bloated sea-lions surrounded by multiple golden greased wrappers.

The first of the month came, and of course, we were both determined to use this first day as a new start. I remember this day so vividly. After having a controlled lunch that consisted of a single meat burger combo instead of my usual double meat, double cheeseburger combo I decided to keep it simple and light to start off the new month. Dinner consisted of a personal veggie pizza instead of my usual large pan meat lovers. I figured that substituting the meat and the large size for a personal veggie pizza was certainly a step up from my "usual." I decided instead of a late-night binge, to go for a walk and shoot some hoops, and since Tone was also once a pretty great basketball player and a great challenge for me that maybe I should invite him, so we could start this new fresh month on the right foot– I approached his door and knocked.

"What up dawg!?" I said from the other side of the closed door.

Tone didn't answer, but I knew he was home, so I walked in slowly.

I saw Tone in bed in a pitch-black room. I noticed in place of his girl was a torn-up large pizza box eaten clean with no sign of a single crumb. *Could it have been from a previous night?* I thought and hoped. But I knew that it couldn't have, as his room reeked of a fresh large meat lover's pizza. I nodded in disappointment, as I knew he fucked up for the day, but unfortunately fucking up had been all too common in our tenure of living together, so I was not surprised as I lightly tapped Tone on the shoulder.

"Umm, what is it?" Tone said groggily.

"You want to shoot hoops dawg?" I asked.

"Nah, Duke. I'm going to recover from this pizza shit." Tone said without budging.

"Cool man, if you change your mind you know where I'm at," I said knowing damn well he would never show.

After about a 20-minute shoot around, all I could think of was why Tone and I could never get out this rut of always fucking up our diets. Whether it be the first of the month, New Year's, a brand spanking new Monday, or the rare first of the month that started on a Monday, we were destined to crash and burn. Considering Tone had most likely already thrown the white flag 20 minutes into his commitment to start the month right, I knew that my time was about to come to submit to a *Whataburger* after this short shoot-around. My original plan was to shoot baskets for at least a good hour, and then go home and simply fall asleep, and conquer day one moving onto day two with confidence. Instead, thoughts of Tone fucking up by eating that large pizza consumed me, so why not fuck up also? After all, starting on the second day of the month was just as good, as long as I got started.

While shooting free-throws which I'm proud to say I would make 18 out of 20, the beautiful lit *Whataburger* sign cast somewhat of a glow just above the backboard perfectly accenting the background of my vision– it was glorious. I looked at my watch, and knew I couldn't fool myself, and was looking forward to a deuce combo with a side of pancakes to conclude the night. I would take a half-court shot completely air balling, as my ball rolled to the bumper of my car. I was never so excited to airball in my life, because I knew I was about to slam dunk a great late-night meal and fall asleep happy and determined to start my diet; except instead of it being on the first of the month, it was the second of the month which in my mind had a nice ring to it.

*I pull along the drive-thru of my local Whataburger anxiously and ordered.*

*"Yes, may* **WE** *have your #2 double meat cheeseburger combo, with a breakfast on a bun sandwich, and an order of pancakes, please?*

*"Do you want to "Whatasize" your combo, and do you want bacon or sausage with your breakfast on a bun?" the drive-through attendant asked.*

*"Yes, please Whatasize, and can you add both the sausage and bacon to the breakfast sandwich? I'll pay the additional charge."*

*"No problem."*

# RECLUSE

*A* WEEK PASSED, AND I had eaten nothing but *Whataburger,* Chinese, and Mexican platters. I had also gone the entire week without talking to Tone. I started to worry if maybe I offended him by walking into his bedroom unannounced that fateful day for which I had no intention of embarrassing him.

I felt like the walls were closing in. Not only had I fucked up the month royally, but by breaking my commitment that night after shooting hoops, I had also not gone out once, except for visiting family. I wanted to check-in on Tone, but when I passed his bedroom, I never once heard his house music blasting, or the light from the bottom of his door lit, or see Francis come by. I needed fresh air, and I figured, why not break out of this monotony, and get shit faced at *Tio Chuy's* and reestablish this past week with Tone. So, instead of barging in, I knocked on his door.

"Yo man, I was thinking of heading to *Tio Chuy's*; are you in? I asked.

After a long sigh that seemed to have pulsed through the door, Tone finally responded.

"Nah bro, I'm good. I think Francis is going to stop by." Tone said.

It was rare that I heard Tone refer to his girl by her first name; he always just referenced her as "boss" which she was to him in the sincerest form– a fucked up form.

"Bitch" I accidentally whispered aloud.

"What?" Tone said.

"Nothing man. That's cool. If you change your mind, you know where I'm at. I said.

***

I struck out that night, and instead of coming home with a hot piece of ass, I came home with my usual from *Whataburger* with a side of pancakes. Later that night, after taking a massive deuce in the toilet, I stepped out of my room and bumped into Tone outside his bedroom into the hallway. This was the first time since that night I walked into his bedroom with that meat lover's pizza that I had seen him. He appeared haggard with creases on his face from what I presume was a great night sleep. He wore a solid white t-shirt that occupied a combination of mustard stains and dried crusted American cheese.

*He must have eaten a fajita botana? Lucky bastard!* I thought.

"What up dawg? You alright?" I asked.

"I'm good," Tone said.

"Let's catch up bro; it's been a while, but first let me take another shit," I said.

"Cool."

I bombarded the toilet like the U.S. dropping Agent Orange atop Vietnamese villages– the toilet had no chance. I flushed prematurely just so the funk wouldn't marinade in my nostrils. After an exhale from my bombardment, I heard Tone lean against the restroom door nearly startling me to death as I was in mid-wipe when Tone's muffled voice passed through the door.

*Jesus fuck!* I thought.

"Hey man, I'm sorry for standing you up again." Tone said.

"It's all good my man," I said.

"Listen, I haven't been a good friend, but I thought I should let you know that Francis and I called it quits a few days back. She came by today to pick up her shit."

I looked up at the ceiling smiling from ear to ear, as I flushed purposely to give Tone somewhat a subliminal message of what I truly thought of Francis.

"No shit, I'm sorry man," I said appeased by the great news and the pun that was applied.

"I just wanted to figure everything out." Tone said.

"I get it man, I've been there before," I said.

"Thanks, and to be honest, I wanted to go join you tonight but was afraid of running into Francis at *Tio Chuy's*." Tone said.

"Nah, I get it. Don't sweat it."

I washed my hands and exited only to realize Tone was not leaning against the door, but instead was sitting.

"Oh shit, you okay?" I asked almost tripping over Tone's shoulder.

"Let me ask you man. Are you afraid of running into your ex's?" Tone asked.

"No, I never really thought about it. If I run into them, I run into them, to be honest," I said.

"Come on man, how much do you weigh now like 240-250?" Tone asked.

"Yeah, so."

"Well, aren't you worried about running into someone, maybe not an ex, but an old buddy from high school, or something?" Tone asked.

"No, what are you trying to get at?" I asked.

"So, them seeing you stretching a 3XL when back in the days you were "cheese" as shit doesn't give you cause to pause as they see you at your physically all-time worse?" Tone said pissed off.

"Dude, if I run into anyone that shit never crosses my mind," I said.

Tone was trying to get to something, I just wasn't sure what he was getting at, but I certainly was curious, and beginning to have some kind of unidentified self-doubt."

"What are you getting at?" I said frustrated.

"Let's say you go to *Tio Chuy's* and you run into Lauren, Ana, Julie or one of your randoms from when you were in shape. You don't think that they would think "Oh my God, I fucked this fat fuck," Tone said sternly.

I recalled running into an old flame from high school when I was at my then blubbery apex. I squirmed, and chills crept through my body as I slid down the wall to sit next to Tone on top our cold white tile defeated.

"Now that I think about it, I did run into an ex a while back."

"And you don't think she had these same thoughts?" Tone asked.

I didn't know what to say as Tone's message was getting much clearer, and his point was getting across. Tone and I talked late into the night continuing our conversation in my bedroom. Tone told me about his fallout with Francis. I did give him my best and most sincere advice about his newly ended relationship. I learned that Francis left Tone not because of some affair of sorts, but because of Tone's ever-expanding waistline. According to Tone she simply told him that "she wasn't attracted to him anymore," and wanted to move on. While Tone broke down crying about their break-up, my mind was stuck on the idea of *What if an old ex saw me as a fat fuck?* Or even worse *what if one of the many girls I fucked over when I was shredded; now sees me as a fat piece of shit?* I thought. It may be narcissistic of me to think this way, but a high sense of insecurity filled my every pore as I somewhat listened to Tone pour his heart out to me.

That night as I lay in bed, I thought that maybe Tone's and Francis' break-up was in some strange way my fault. After all, I was the one that introduced him to plus-size meals while also influencing him to embrace my lethargic lifestyle. Perhaps his warping my mind and becoming self-conscious about running into an ex or old friend was his way of paying me back, which would be well deserved. Oh well, now that Francis was out, maybe he and I could recover from this blown month and focus on getting into shape, and then dominate the dating scene together and rule this world resurrecting the Tre-Tone Experience.

Tone and I went to *Tio Chuy's* one more time throughout our remaining period living together. Sadly, our parameters of going out only consisted of each other's company exclusively downloading a movie, and usually going to a drive-thru killing a *Whataburger*. If we ever did go out, it would be to family functions, and because of our new heightened insecurity, we'd often cancel our appearances eventually creating rifts with beloved family members– all for the sake of a "reclusive" lifestyle. The idea of our weight becoming the topic of conversation at these family occasions was too much for Tone and me to handle considering such an idea would ever occur. Seeing that Tone and I came from great families, and we knew they would never judge us; it just became more about the idea of simply disappointing them by looking at us which by all means was soul crushing.

Luckily for Tone, he plateaued at about 260-pounds for 2 more years. As for Francis, she, of course, would submit to the cliché and hook-up a week after their break-up completely neglecting all those years they were together.

The "recluse" lifestyle for me continued even as I complete this sentence a mere 10 years later. Yes, that's right, about 10 years of my life has been dedicated to burgers and rarely leaving my apartment unless it was absolutely necessary. The simplest of tasks would be difficult, an example being: buying groceries. For me to go out and buy groceries would take tremendous strategy all for the sake of avoiding any possibility of bumping into someone from my past.

I tend to look back from time to time, and before this reclusive concept was realized, I never appreciated how great at life I was at until that fateful night with Tone before he shook up my world. In the process of being a recluse, I lost touch with Tone and the fellas. I mean sure we'd hang-out every now and then but blowing my late 20s and my 30s to bullshit was a crime against life, and I could only pray that somehow, I could one day recoup this decade of shame, and explore life to its fullest all for the sake of making up for time.

> "Yes! Can **WE** order a large pan meat lover's pizza?" I asked the lady over the phone.
> "Sure, if you order 6 buffalo wings, you get a side order of cheese sticks for free. Can I add that to your order?"
> Holy shit! "Yes! **WE'D** like that, thank you." I said.
> "Is there anything else I can add?" the lady working for the pizza joint asked.
> "Can you also add the cheesecake deluxe? That would be all."

# HOOP DREAMS

$\mathcal{M}$Y GREATEST MEMORIES GROWING-UP was coming home from school, rolling up a tortilla and walking to the park to play basketball. On the way to the park, I'd have my tortilla hanging off my lips like a cigar while I'd be practicing my dribbling drills, most specifically, my crossover. While dribbling the ball through my legs, and behind my back, I'd stop by my homeboy's cribs for a mere minute and gather each one by one and play basketball until sundown.

Playing streetball every day of my youth, and well into my 20s, led me to become a pretty good player, even winning the city of McAllen 3-point contest at the age of 19. It was playing on the streets where I gained my ability to not only talk shit but back it up through my play. As a matter of fact, Tone would give me the nickname "Bad-Habit" for my ability to give "facials" to an opponent when he clearly wasn't looking for one. A "facial" is a slang basketball term where someone plays tight defense, and his opponent still drains a long distant shot while the defender's hand is in the shooter's face. The nickname stuck, and to be honest, I felt like I earned it. Who knew my nickname "Bad-Habit" would eventually serve as a double entendre for my eating habits years later.

Now, I rarely played organized ball. Besides playing in a few summer, and AAU leagues, I never had the chance to play for my junior high or high school teams. The reason being that I would flunk out every six weeks, not because I wasn't smart enough to do the work, but because I always skipped school. I even recall my vice principal senior year taking me to her office and telling me that she had never seen so many absences from one student in her 12 years of administration. Looking back, I suppose school basketball wasn't that important to me, and I was fine just being a street-baller.

I had such a great time playing basketball that my crew and I would often travel to neighboring parks and play for bragging rights. One of my fondest memories was traveling to Corpus Christi with my squad to play a pick-up game 150 miles away—which I'm proud to say we won handily.

Eventually, my street-ball "career" came to a halt when I fell on my ankle playing a pick-up game of basketball. It would be months after my ankle injury that I'd play again, and when I did, I was never the same. Whenever I'd go in for a rebound or lay-up, I'd always fear to fall on my ankle again leading me to play with caution and no aggression, which was never my nature causing me to feel like a neutered dog. Because my mind was fucking with me, I would eventually put the basketball away and focus full time on my San Antonio Spurs, and dream of one day replacing Coach Popovich and become one of the greatest coaches in NBA history, but I suppose being the 2000 City of McAllen 3-point champ is good enough.

\*\*\*

One thing about being a street-baller is rarely playing in a basketball gym. I admit, whenever I played in an indoor court, I became unstoppable because I knew it was a privilege to play in such a magical wooden space, that I ALWAYS wanted to play my best. Not to mention, there was no wind factor which was a major plus especially for an all-time great shooter like me.

I had just moved back to my parent's home. I had weighed about 265-pounds, and I knew I had to do something about my weight. Now, remember, before I began gaining my weight back I used to run about 8-12 miles a day with ease. So, now that I was on the fast track to 300-pounds, I knew there was no way I could ever go back to running 8-12 miles again especially as a 265-pound man. I had to ease into it.

I didn't want to start running again, because I didn't want to endure the monotony of running from point A to point B. So, *what was I going to do? I had to do something?* I realized that it had been a while since I last played basketball, I believe the last time I played was when I was playing by myself when I lived with Tone and chucked that half-court shot. I thought, *yeah that's it, I'll play some ball.* Playing basketball was perfect. I could ease into it by shooting jumpers to regain my shot back, and eventually build-up the endurance to play basketball like I used to when I was a kid.

***

First thing in the morning I drove to the closest basketball court to my parents' house and began shooting for the first time in over a year. I believe out of my first fifteen shots I made one, so to say I was rusty was an understatement. I took another shot, and the ball would bounce off the rim ricocheting to the other side of the court causing me to move more than I wanted to. Ten minutes into shooting, and I was beginning to lose interest because I couldn't hit a damn shot to save my life. So, as I grabbed the rebound from my own bad shot, I purposely shoot a five-footer, so I could feel the ball go through the hoop hoping psychologically I could turn the corner and make some damn shots—shooting a "gimmie" like that five-footer is a shooting trick to help the player refocus and regain confidence in his or her shot. I grabbed my made rebound and quickly turn for another "gimmie" when suddenly I hear from afar "Yo!" Distracted, I air-balled the five-footer and turned my attention towards the yelling. I grabbed my ball, and it was an old man shouting for my attention. "Hey man! We're short a player, you want to come and play with us?" I would shout "Yes!" without hesitation. *I was about to play in a gym*, I couldn't even recall when the last time I played indoors. I jogged to the gym trying to remain calm when in reality my enthusiasm was beginning to get the best of me.

I entered the gym, and it was glorious. I stood at the entrance and thanked Dr. Naismith for creating heaven on Earth—I do the sign of the cross and exhaled thankful for being blessed to have such an opportunity to play in such a space—I was in Mecca. I slowly bounced my ball onto the wooden floor and hear that sweet vibrato rumble off my eardrums causing me to become flushed with goosebumps. There were five men who appeared to be in their late 40s shooting around, and because of my respect for the court and my opponents, I dribbled aside the corner 3-point line waiting for the man who called me in to introduce me.

A minute had passed when finally, the older man would introduce himself.

"I'm Dr. Garza and your name?" Dr. Garza would extend his hand for a handshake.

"Tre."

"Let me introduce you to the guys." We approached the free throw line.

"Guys this is Tre, and he's going to make us even."

I waved while hugging my ball in front of my gut.

"This is Dr. Reyes."

The older guys looked me up and down and probably assessed that I'd be too out of shape to play. I must be honest; although they were in great shape, I knew they couldn't hang with me. As I shook Dr. Reyes hand, he must've been 6'3 a hundred pounds soaking wet.

"Nice to meet you," I said.

Dr. Garza would introduce me to the other three geriatrics who were both also doctors by the name of Dr. Rivera, Dr. Diaz, and Dr. Cortes who were all just a bit taller than me but weren't shit.

As we warmed up, I took evaluation as I mostly worked on my dribbling instead of shooting because I wanted to access what I was up against. Considering, that these men were much older than I, they were fantastic players. I could immediately tell that they probably played every weekend for which I knew I was in for a good challenge especially because I've been out of the game for a while.

After warm-ups, we shot free-throws to decide teams. The first three to make the free-throws would be on one team and the others who missed would be the other. Strange enough, the first three to shoot free-throws made their shots including myself as I was pleased my basketball absence hadn't affected my shot. Then again, I was in a gym.

I was teamed up with Dr. Garza, Dr. Rivera, and decided to play full-court. Now, granted I hadn't played full-court much less basketball in years, so I knew it was going to be a test of endurance and mental fortitude, but I was up for the challenge.

Before the start of the game, Dr. Rivera tells me to guard their point guard Dr. Cortes; who out of the three was the shortest, and because I was the shortest on my team, I supposed it was a natural pairing. Two dribbles from inbounding, I knew he didn't have the best handle as he dribbled with an open stance. The ball was completely exposed for a steal, so I decided to play him close. Immediately, I stopped him in his tracks just after he crossed the half-court. In desperation, Dr. Cortes heaves the ball from over his head to his teammate on the far-left hash-mark almost tossing it out of bounce. I would leach onto my opponent never giving him an inch. Considering he was in much better shape than I and was obviously much faster, he couldn't shake me loose. Because he couldn't get open, his teammate was forced to chuck the ball from the hash-mark missing the entire backboard causing my teammate Dr. Rivera to shout "AIRBALL!"

Since I was defending their point guard, Dr. Cortes, I suppose I was our point guard as Dr. Rivera inbounded the ball to me. I brought the ball up court, and Dr. Cortes decides to "attempt" to lock me up defensively. As he closes to full-court press me, I smile, and quickly cross the ball over through my right leg and burn him right leading him to fall face first as I rushed up the court leaving him behind. Now, I wasn't as fast as I used to be, so he was able to chase me from behind. I would cross half-court with Dr. Cortes by my side, except his defense had relaxed as I assumed he had respect for my game because I knew what I was doing with the ball. I pulled up to the top of the 3-point key and asked for a screen by waving in Dr. Garza. Dr. Garza immediately sets me up for what should've been a pick and roll, but I wanted to show these old fogies that I was a killer. The screen was set. I dribbled right, as Dr. Garza sprinted towards the basket with his hand up wide-open looking for me to lob him the ball for the easy lay-up. Instead, I pulled up from the center arc of the 3-point line and shoot. The ball had a perfect rotation as my arm and hand stayed frozen in the air. Everyone, including my teammates' heads, followed the arc of the ball resembling the broadest of rainbows—SWISH! I was back, and there was nothing these old geriatrics could do, as I'm sure they judged me because of my fat ass. While backpedaling towards half-court, I purposely leave my arm up and hand in the same pose as my three-point shot.

Dr. Cortes would bring the ball back up court and once again his open stance lures me to press him again. Naturally, Cortes stops and pulls the ball up over his head looking for either Dr. Diaz or Reyes. It was the fear in his eyes when I decided to swipe the ball from his grip and tip it over his head. I rushed around him nearly falling onto my knees trying to get the steal. I get in front of him and put my newly fat ass to box him out and possess the ball racing across the court to score. It's in this fast break as I tried to break away for the easy layup when "IT" happens. Although it was the third play of the game, I admit I was already huffing and puffing, but when I finally got that steal racing my way to the basket my back felt this insane tightness causing me to pull-up and dribble out as I waited for both Dr. Garza and Rivera to catch-up. While dribbling, I hunched over to stretch my back trying to appear like nothing was wrong. My back felt like it was being held by a string as the discomfort was barely tolerable enough to finish the game.

I would lag the entire game. I could no longer run with Dr. Cortes often switching with their Center Dr. Diaz, so I could not move as much, which didn't matter because they both would be scoring on me at will. Also, because I was designated point-guard no matter what the tempo of the game was, I was forced to slow it down and walk towards the half-court stretching my back while walking and wiggling my torso like I was a dog standing on its hind legs. Thankfully, my crossover the second play of the game earned me the respect to allow Dr. Cortes to play off me, as I was able to bring up the ball freely. Every time, I'd pass the half-court I'd immediately pass it off and stay on top of the key and wait with my hands on my knees stretching my back for comfort. I could tell I was pissing off my teammates as I assumed they thought I wasn't in pain but rather out of shape which I was, but in this case, my back was the problem.

We'd end up getting blown out losing 21 to 10, as the game turned out to be more of a 2 on 3 situation. Because I was forced to stand still offensively being completely ineffective, I realize I was more suited for today's NBA game where it's okay to just stand and shoot. I took 6 shots in the game making 2 three-pointers and allowing the other team to score on me freely like James Harden playing defense.

After the game they wanted to play another, but I would make a quick excuse that I had to get going, but in reality, I wanted to hit the showers and hang my head in defeat and curse to myself *that my weight gain caused my back to fuck up, or else I would've killed those guys.*

This would be the first time when I realized that gaining weight could throw off your entire body as silly as that may sound. I spent that night in searing back pain not able to afford to see a doctor. I would double down on painkillers praying to God that I'd wake-up good to go in the morning, but also drown myself in sugary sports drinks and my usual number 2 from *Whataburger.* As my eyelids began to weigh down that night, I knew basketball was over, and all I had left were my hoop dreams.

# THE MAN IN BLACK

*L*IFE AS AN OBESE man can be a bit repetitive. Now, when you weigh 350-pounds fashion tends to leave you behind never giving a fuck. This is when repetition occurs in the saddest of forms. Now, we large people fall into the idea that wearing black is "slimming," and although true, we know in actuality that we more resemble Shamu on his worst of days, as 2 or 3 solid black t-shirts are on heavy rotation.

As for me, Monday, Tuesday, and Wednesday required one black t-shirt with my favorite blue gym shorts to be worn to exhaustion. Thursday, Friday, and Saturday another black t-shirt with my red gym shorts finish the week leaving Sunday for a wash day where I'd sport clothes from my previous size; in this case for when I was 25-pounds lighter and the chance for my shorts ripping was an extreme possibility. Now, there are many large men that can pull off the "snug" look, and I respect that tremendously, but that one hour where I'm waiting for my clothes to dry was rather an inconvenience as the "snug" life wasn't for me.

Of course, what do I do when it comes to a formal situation? During this period of my life I had been living at home for many years now, and since I had left Tone's apartment which then I weighed about 260ish, I had now crossed the 350-pound barrier and even worse was wearing a 5XL.

The formal occasion was my niece's baptismal that was about 2 months away. Now, my plan of course, was to lose crazy weight in those two-months so that I could have more options to wear something decent besides something black and grease stained. Unfortunately, I was once again having a love affair with *Jack-in-the-box's* double bacon cheeseburger amongst other things, so the odds of following through with my 2-month diet plan was close to impossible. Now, for most people, they would've put love in front of personal destruction. An example of this would be a person telling himself "lose weight for your niece, if you really love her you would do it," which all sounds motivational, but the way my mind was at the time, those thoughts were never a concept, or never once crossed my mind. Unfortunately, greased bags were more important, and even as I write this sentence, I'm considering going on a late-night *Whataburger* run.

***

The event was fast approaching, and the idea of losing weight was long gone. By this time, I was looking for a place with nice clothes for large men. I knew they didn't make button-up shirts my size in department stores, so I figured maybe I'd find a nice clean *Polo* shirt somewhere soon.

Two-weeks until the big day, and I was in panic mode. After a midday afternoon snack consisting of two large bowls of *Fruity Pebbles*, it hit me like a bolt of lightning. *Why not check-out Wal-Mart?* I thought.

Of course, I was in full recluse mode and scheduled in my mind that I'd go around 4 in the morning where the odds of running into someone from my "skinny" days would be near impossible. *Wal-Mart* had to be it. I'd seen all the insensitive videos of fellow "gargantuans" perusing through the aisles like well-organized herds; surely, they'd appeal to their demographic and have mega plus-sized shirts– I couldn't wait.

I walked into the "Mecca" with my eyes lit with deep anticipation. I quickly made my way towards the clothing department directly to the rack of folded up *Polo* shirts. As I perused through the sized stickers labeled on each shirt, I scroll directly to the plus sizes. "3XL, 4XL, 5XL." Now, granted I wasn't aware of my size at the time. I had been rocking the same two black t-shirts for about 2 years now, so the 5XL that I currently wore must have stretched out its fabric to its final thread, so maybe these 5XLs weren't the 5XLs that I needed. Then again, the 5XLs I had always worn weren't stretched, and maybe, just maybe I've lost inches to where I could fit into a smaller T. I grabbed a navy blue 5XL, and a red 4XL *Polo* shirt in hopes that they would both fit considering the navy blue resembled a black *Polo* shirt.

I approached the dressing room, and two rooms were open. The first room I opened seemed to have been built for some skinny ass mother-fucker. The seat that occupied that room would never have been large enough to even cover one of my ass cheeks.

*Fuck that!* I thought.

I looked into the other dressing room, and it was fit for a Roman Emperor with a bench resembling one from a baseball dugout. I proudly tossed the shirts onto the corner of the bench. I lifted my faded solid black t-shirt over my head, and what seemed to be years in the making and as hard as it was to believe, I saw myself in the mirror for the first time without a t-shirt in years.

Before, when I stepped out of the shower sure I'd see my body, but in all actuality, it was as if I looked past the mirror and only focused on my locks of hair– which was my best feature, but never looked fully into the mirror. So, as I stood there gawking in the dressing room mirror, it was as if I was staring at a complete stranger. All I could really do was nod my head in disappointment and realize that I destroyed the only thing that was truly mine and was God-given.

I took a deep breath and grabbed the red 4XL solid *Polo* shirt. I held it against my chest and knew instantly by looking into the mirror that there was no way that it was going to fit. *Fuck-it,* I thought and slipped it on. The only problem was that it barely went past my man tits. I rolled down the residual shirttail as much as possible, and of course, it was snug. I began to sweat beads. I tossed the 4XL towards the corner of the king bench and took another deep breath as I grabbed the 5XL pissed. Something was telling me that there was no way possible that the 5XL would ever fit because the one size smaller was so snug on me, I mean how much of a difference would one more size be? Upon sizing up the 5XL in front of the mirror, I commenced in a small prayer, and as I wiped my brow in anticipation and hopefulness, I would catch my breath. I slid over the shirt, and it felt nice amongst my shoulders, and as I rolled it over on top of my man-tits, and my bulbous gut the *Polo* shirt barely past my belly button 3 inches shy of covering the bottom of my "front-ass." Pissed, I took off the shirt in one quick lashing and sat on the dressing room bench disappointed and drenched in sweat resembling one of those athletes after a disappointing defeat. I turned to look at my obese "womanly" figure in the mirror wanting to go berserk over what I did to God's gift. *What did I do to deserve this fucking curse?* I thought. For some reason, I recalled a memory from a few years back when I was driving home, and nearly had a car accident all because I wanted to avoid hitting a large turtle trying to cross the road. I never understood why this near-death experience was important to me, and why it always seemed to resonate with me whenever I had a bad moment such as me trying on fucking clothes. After I had straightened out my car, I looked into the rearview mirror and saw a large truck weaving through traffic and purposely running over the turtle, crushing it into a bloody shell soup. I still recall seeing blood splatter from my fleeting car. Needless to say, I was shocked when I saw the truck go out of his way to make this turtle road-kill, but what put the cherry-on-top of this *moment* was when the truck caught up to me. I would see the man in the truck laughing carelessly with some dime-ass girl. All I could think of was *that this cocksucka just committed murder and he was going to go home in about 5 minutes and get laid? Are you kidding me? He received the benefit of tossing a dime-piece while being a dick, and I was forced to be stuck in this dressing room disappointed that I'm going to let down my niece–* FUCK *THAT!* I had never told anyone about that memory about the turtle because I knew it was my way of blaming outside forces for my cataclysmic dietary fall.

I thought of ways to get out of my niece's baptismal while sitting on the king bench defeated. This would be the exact *moment* in my life where I contemplated suicide for the first time ever. After all, I was in a store with an infinite amount of pills just two aisles over, and access to a gun rack one section away. In all seriousness, as I sat there glistening from simply trying on two fucking shirts, I looked at my reflection and envisioned my family looking for me at the baptismal making my sister and niece's big day all about me. Suddenly, buying a fuck load of pills didn't sound so bad after all, and seemed like a peaceful way to go out. Imagine finally having a way to end my curse of constant thoughts of food and diet.

Now my tears corresponded with the beads of sweat drizzling from my brow as I shook nervously as suicide was sincerely becoming an option. While gawking at my astounding reflection, my heartfelt crushed, not only because I would let everyone down by not showing up to the baptismal, but if I decided to end things now the idea of my father and mother standing over my grave was by far more crushing than I could ever imagine. Thoughts of *why can't I say no to my dumbass ways? Why am I so fucking weak? And why does it have to be so damn hard?* I grabbed the red 4XL *Polo* shirt, and wiped my sweat and tears out of frustration, and tossed it aside, and then grabbed the 5XL and suddenly stretched the living shit out of it praying that it would stretch a half inch over my gut. Like Clark Kent tearing apart his suit to turn into Superman, for me, it was like I was tearing this shirt to save my life. I needed this shirt to stretch as much as possible to fit; I just needed it to happen.

After I stretched the shirt as much as possible without tearing it, I put the shirt down to catch my breath and grabbed the 4XL again to wipe the sweat dripping from the back of my hair appearing as if I just came out of a shower. I held the 5XL against my obese womanly body, and like a rookie fresh out the minor leagues holding that infamous pen stripped Yankee uniform for the first time, I cried. I just knew it was going to fit, as I must have stretched it two more sizes to an unflattering 6 or 7XL. I tried on the shirt, and it fit comfortably. I sat back down on the bench running my fingers through my perspired long hair and smiled. As I checked out at *Wal-Mart,* I made the conscious decision to buy the 4XL as well, in hopes that one day I get my shit together and fit into the shirt instead of using it as a sweat rag.

***

The day of the baptismal I woke-up late and realized my family left for the event without me. The night before, I drank myself into a drunken stupor that led to a legendary night of *Whataburger* that I wasn't aware of ever ordering. When I woke up there were numerous wrappers surrounding my mattress like stones from a massive Indian burial ground. I was grateful my parents left without me because it meant that I could take my time and get in uniform without the rush of my ma shouting through my door "LET'S GO! WE CAN'T BE LATE!" Besides, my mom is a truly great person in all forms of the word, and one of her greatest qualities that I wish I had was her punctuality. If I'm not mistaken, in her 25 years of being a teacher, she was never late a single day, which was something I could only aspire to do.

I rolled out of bed and noticed I had about 45 minutes to get to the baptismal a town away in Edinburg, Texas. Sadly, because McAllen has no cross-town highway, everyone is forced to go through mad traffic to get anywhere, causing you to take at least forty-five minutes to get where you needed to be. Needless to say, it is frustrating beyond words. I sat up on the side of the bed, collected the golden wrappers, and what apparently was two completely empty 32-ounce sodas. Of course, I could've just read the receipt in the bag, but it was like a bad note left behind from a one-night stand that coincidently I used to leave all the time for my "randoms" back in my glory days before I discovered "Fast Food Alley." Judging by the length of the receipt, I knew without looking that it could not have been good. Besides, my gut felt so bulbous and like a stone that the golden wrappers weren't the only evidence of my shitty night.

After I dropped last night's deuce, I grabbed the 5XL which I hadn't worn since that near-fatal night. I suddenly recalled my sister telling me a few weeks ago which led to that night at *Wal-Mart* that "I better wear something nice!" Of course, because my sister is the patriarch of my family, we're all supposed to just sit and abide. As much as I'd love to say, "No problem," to wearing something nice, unfortunately, I couldn't abide. I wish there was a way I could somehow make my sister and others realize what us morbidly obese folk physically, and emotionally endure by having them understand that our options of simply wearing some-thing "nice" at times are almost impossible without resorting to fancying a bed-sheet, or even worst the same-old black t-shirt with 2-year-old grease stains. Is it an excuse? Of course, but like alcoholism, and drug addiction, obesity is an addiction, and one of the most unrecognized and paralyzing symptoms of obesity is "self-reflection" especially when it comes to public appearances.

Now for the sake of my niece, I would love to rock a 3-piece suit with plenty of room to dance (fitted clothing,) rather than to submit to the "obese clichéd uniform" of growing the fat man's pubic patched beard just to give the illusion of hiding my many numerous chin rolls. Another piece of the "obese uniform" is growing your hair, and for me letting my lengthy hair grow past my neck to cover-up as much face as possible allowed me to get through the day without being recognized. Most importantly you "skinny folk" should understand that we would do anything to wear something "nice," but most importantly wish we didn't have this self-inflicted burden. The simple fact is that we know that we look like shit, and we just want you to understand that we already know that we let you down by appearing this way, and more than likely beat ourselves up because we didn't dress to your reasonable standard. We just want you to understand why.

***

The baptismal went accordingly, besides the obvious countless eyes ogling my monstrous size accompanied by nods of disappointment, and whispers about me such as "Jesus, look at that guy." Or my all-time favorite "Move, so he can squeeze through," which was often met with chuckles or pissed-off grins. Either, or, when I go out in public, this is the norm. I don't expect anyone to feel sorry for me as we don't look for empathy; rather we hope that you simply understand. Authors say, that "we write for an audience of one," but for me, the reason why I'm writing this is not only for you to understand what us large people are going through, but know that our addiction is just as valid as any other. As much as I'd love to say "no" to a burger, some kind of chemical reaction fucks with my mind and taste buds leading me to fiend for a burger as if I had no control, while also leading to additional side meals on the same order. Also, like any other addiction, we also hurt our loved ones, as our addiction often leads us to a life of solitude and dismay except we can't cover our tracks with a long sleeve shirt or avoid our hot-spots for a few weeks to get sober and get a clean shave from a haggard addictive exterior. Imagine us "plus-sizers" putting on a shirt and magically appearing average weight. After all, a black shirt and vertical striping can only do so much; instead, what you see is what you get.

# THE BUMP INTO

*L*IFE SEEMS TO PUNCH you in the gut when you're least expecting it. For most people, it usually occurs when family emergencies happen or unexpected job loss before Christmas happens, and believe me I've had my versions as well. I'm just thankful and hopeful that they never occur again or at least for decades to come.

Although life can hit you swiftly, when it comes to a large man, one of the most common occurrences comes in the form of what I call the "bump into." Now sure, I stole this term from the greatest sitcom of all-time *Seinfeld,* but the term "bump into" is appropriate for such an occasion. So, what is the "fat man's" version of a "bump into? Well, it's exactly what it means. It's when you bump into someone you much rather not bump into because one: you are either losing at life or two or in my case the last time I saw this person I was in a much better physical state. Now, the life of a large man, we understand that "bump-into's" are simply a part of life.

Unfortunately, we must eat, or else we die which for most of us is a valid and much often taken attempt. So, besides hitting drive-thrus where we could avoid getting down and running into a familiar foe, at times, we must step out of our car and risk being seen all for the sake of our addiction.

For me, I had many "bump into's;" after a near decade of the "plus-size" life you are doomed to experience such discomfort all for the sake of not being rude. Now, this "bump into" was the worst version any large person could ever endure, and that was bumping into an old flame or ex.

By this time in my life, I was years into my reclusive state and made my expanding habit by living in the drive-thru lanes, and strategically shopping at our local *H-E-B* Superstore well past midnight, where I knew the odds of a "bump into" were close to none. This day was memorable to me because it was a few days before my favorite holiday which predictably is Thanksgiving. Now, I made my wonderful mom a deal that in addition to making the turkey that she would also make her glorious ham for which I was willing to pay for. The only problem was that my mom wanted to go during their peak hours, in which I knew that I would have to get out of my mom's car and risk breaking my "reclusiveness," and risk a "bump into" for the sake of a ham. I began to think *maybe the ham isn't all that important, or maybe I could give her the cash,* and *I'll wait in the car.* Unfortunately, my mom was adamant that I go inside with her so she could spend time with her "oldest son" as she so eloquently put it. Thoughts flooded through my mind on how I was going to let her down even to the point of asking her to cancel the ham altogether. But the thoughts were soon overwhelmed by her immaculate ham "pimp slapping" my taste buds into oblivion, as I knew there was no way I could go another year without her ham. The obese idiot in me was willing to risk it all and join my mom in a "mother-son" adventure at our local superstore in hopes that she wouldn't witness a potential cataclysmic beat down of any confidence I may have had left because of a possible "bump into." To say I wasn't about to endure a session of nervous perspiration would simply be a lie.

Now, the mind of a morbidly obese man that has built a life of reclusivity does everything on strategy Is it exhausting? Of course, beyond any man's imagination, but it is absolutely necessary, at least for me. Now, there are many large people that don't give a fuck, and for those I give kudos to, but for me who was once a male dime-piece (at least I like to think so) had become to vain to ever walk the aisles of anywhere comfortably all while weighing 300, 350, or 400-pounds, not to say that life in the 200s is all that easy. Believe me, I remember those days, and they sucked, but I'll take 299-pounds any day of the week over any weight past 300, especially 400.

As I walked through the aisles with my mom, my eyes were 10 aisles ahead scanning for a potential "bump into" leaving any form of decent conversation extremely vague and usually ending with "ah huh, yeah, or my favorite, "sure." Mom would eventually go her own way as I would predictably peruse the candy section. Now, I was rocking my outstretched famed, faded grease stained Monday-Wednesday black t-shirt hoping that the tail of the shirt didn't expose any butt-crack what-so-ever. A few minutes perusing through the candy aisle, I pulled down my shirt to cover any form of exposure as I reached for the gummy *Coke Haribos*. As I extended my shooting arm to the highest extent for those damn gummy *Cokes*, that's when "IT" happened.

"Tre, is that you?" in the tone of what I imagine would be an angel. Beads of sweat instantly formed, and without having to turn to see who was calling my name, I knew exactly who it was. My heart rate surpassed 200 beats a minute, as I turned slowly with a pursed grin.

"Lauren, hey!"

I hadn't seen Lauren since we had broken up nearly 12 years ago when my beginning weight with her started at 160 and ended at 282-pounds after many years together. She looked phenomenal as if God kept her this pristine just so I could experience this ass-kicking that I was currently enduring– thank God Mom wasn't there to witness it. I would scan the aisle hoping Mom wouldn't walk through to witness her son get destroyed when Lauren's pure smile would lure me in. My mind began to race to figure out how I could reverse time and miraculously weigh a 160- pounds just so I could make Lauren look at me like the man she once dated over a decade ago, instead of the obese person that I currently was– I reached in for a hug.

"Oh my Goodness Tre, how have you been?" Lauren asked with somewhat of a victorious chuckle, causing my head to turn like my old dog the late great Casper the G.O.A.T.

Thoughts of *if I was in shape when this bump into occurred* would shuffle through my mind while thinking *let's get back together and engage in an innocent rendezvous.* But those thoughts would be obliterated by the idea that she must be astonished by what she was looking at, and because of her "spectacle" eyes, it was clear that she thought that she beat me in life or couldn't believe she was with such a fat fuck.

The small talk continued, and as improbable as it may be, the only way I could've salvaged this horrendous "bump into" was if some kind of "stick-up" occurred just so I could save her life, but knowing my luck if that happened I'd most likely roll my ankle falling directly on top of her, or even worse have the thug shoot her while I dove out of the way using her as a shield which would be most probable, in this improbable situation. As she kept talking, I on the other hand just stood there taking the hit as the back of my head became saturated with sweat. I made sure to pull my shirt collar away from my neck to make sure that no sweat ring formed.

Surprisingly, I learned that she was single with no kids, all but confirming that if I was halfway decent then I would have certainly slammed her for "old time's sake." I also learned that she became a dentist, and as a matter of fact, she gave me her card to set an appointment which I knew, and she knew would never happen. The thought of her digging into my sugar impacted molars all while reminiscing about the good 'old days would be a nightmare.

I wasn't sure if this "bump into" made her feel like she won. I mean, after all, it's been 12 years. I'm sure she'd never thought of me once since our break-up, and maybe that's what I deserved. Although I never saw judgment in her eyes from this brief encounter, I was more absolved by her ageless beauty and my cryptic thoughts. I was okay with her defeating me because she looked happy and radiant beyond measure, and as we said our goodbyes and she walked away, my pursed smile soon loosened, and I was able to smile proudly that I once was with a girl, now woman that turned out ahead in life.

I put away the *Coke* gummies, overwhelmed with unexplainable emotions as I wiped my brow of sweat. I joined my mom in the pay-out counter and saw Lauren walking the aisles from afar as I envisioned one day I'd have another bump into with her, except, I'd be the version that could stand-up to her as we'd both greet each other in victory.

# BECOMING A NINJA

$\mathcal{M}$Y LIFE AT THIS point was not only physically but emotionally and certainly mentally exhausting. I mean, for Christ's sake if I wanted to simply go to the corner store just to fill up my tank of gas, I would go at times where the odds of bumping into an ex-was close to none and usually well past midnight. This was for everything: including movies, hanging out with old homeboys or simply picking up fast-food. Everything I did that required going outside was met with the instant thought of *if I'm going to leave the house, I can't be seen.* Did I ever get seen upon strategy? Of course, especially when one of my homeboys insisted that we go out for some late night "feed your beer munchies," and for my homeboys and me *Whataburger* was where it was at, and that went for anyone who lived in the Rio Grande Valley much less the entire population of Texas. The odds of a "bump into" were certainly possible. Now, whether that was an ex or an old friend they were both something I did not want to experience especially after my bout with Lauren.

Normally, I made up some bull-shit to get out of such a possible situation no matter how great of a time I could have with my boys. Like emphasizing which *Whataburger* to go to when in actuality I knew it would be less packed, and the odds of a "bump into" weren't possible. I'd even go as far as offering to drive if it meant going two towns over to simply sit comfortably and enjoy what would most likely be my second burger of the day. It would often work; as a matter of fact, it always worked especially when I offered my driving services. Although going two towns over meant that the night was going to come to a close whichever *Whataburger* I chose, it was more important that I eat in peace without the constant stress of a possible "bump into," and I'm proud to say that I don't ever recall having a meaningful "bump into" in all those years hanging with my homeboys.

To this day I'm still enduring my "reclusive" stage thanks to Tone. I hung out with my homeboys far and in-between making it a point to miss out on big occasions. I would and still go out of my way to make-up some bull-shit so I could get out of them like: "I have to visit my "abuela," but I'll make-it-up to you when I get back." Those "make-up" dates only occurred on a Sunday because I knew no one would go to a bar on a Sunday much less a Sunday night. I knew the people I grew up with were so insecure with how "it would look," that they would rather be at church and post pictures on *Facebook* than be at a bar on a Sunday afternoon for the sake of being aesthetically appropriate.

Another variation of "becoming a Ninja" was sneaking out of my parents' home just to pick up a food order all while in my thirties. Now, I was used to going out whenever I wanted and picking-up a grand slam order and bingeing in front of a movie or T.V. show. After my father's business closed, and I moved back home, my father ridiculed me every time I walked in with food, especially after just finishing dinner or lunch an hour earlier. With his judgmental eyes and along with his long-winded sighs of disappointment it became a bit too much. I knew he wasn't malicious of any sort; as a matter of fact, I knew he knew I was miserable and he just wanted me to be happy and healthy. So, to avoid disappointing Mom and Dad I forced myself to wait until 2 or 3 at night to sneak out of my house like I was a teenager again, but instead of getting pussy, I settled for the deluxe ground beef patties every night. It became a ritual, a ritual of survival and gluttony. Interestingly enough, my daytime meals were sensible unless I knew no one would be home that day in which I went into "berserk mode" and ate like it was my last meal. During the weekdays I would wait until midnight for a late-night binge where I'd strategize for what I was about to gorge myself into. In all seriousness, my tongue would salivate like *Marvels'* comic character Venom. I couldn't wait until my parents called it a night and fell asleep, so I could hit the streets.

So, this was my nightly strategy. My parents normally went to bed around 11:30 p.m. sometimes at midnight. I would wait more than just an hour so I knew that they would at least be in a deep sleep or wait until the light under the door was off, so I could tip-toe out of the house hoping and praying to God that the unlocking of the front door wouldn't wake them, especially my dad. Did they know I was up to no good? Of course, but for me, it gave me some assurance that I could get away with something so self-destructive that I couldn't wait to do it again the following night.

Now, there were times when I'd go out to pick up some food for a late night "sloth session" that I wouldn't be able to go inside the house, because a light could be seen from my front door in which I always made sure that all the lights would be off as an indicator for such an occasion. When the light was on, I knew someone was awake. I would wait in the car for 5 minutes knowing damn well that I would never walk in knowing my Dad was awake in the living room and have him see me with nearly half a dozen greased bags. The disappointment on his face was far worse than when he saw my high school report card back in the days.

Seeing lights on after I arrived home occurred on several occasions enabling me to develop my ninja skills further. So, when the lights were on and 5 minutes had passed, I knew I had to do something or risk my food getting cold. Now, I know most people would be thinking "Dude, just eat in your car." Well, sadly I was in a stage in my life where I was so paranoid about eating in my car and having a way to improbable "bump into." Just the image of an old-flame knocking on my car window while inhaling a deuce from *Whataburger* would destroy me beyond recognition; just writing this sentence gives me the chills.

While I sat there as the time ticked by, and the lights still burned through the window door like early rise of the morning sun, instead of walking in with a bundle of grease bags and getting caught like a robber, I decided to put the food in the trunk just in case my dad tried to play me and wanted to check my car. I could only imagine opening my trunk and seeing my "habit" sitting there on top the tire iron like a dead body, and Dad nod in disappointment or even worse nods and grins unsurprisingly.

I decided to go in, and when I opened the front door, there was no one in sight. Strangely enough, whenever I'd be in such an occasion, there was never a person in sight. In retrospect, I now believe it was my dad's indicator that he knew I was up to no good and that he was most importantly thinking of me. Knowing what I know now I wish I knew this then, maybe I would've tossed the bags, but of course, that was never going to happen. When I made my rounds and confirmed no one was awake, I shut the lights off again and hauled ass to my trunk to get the food and rushed through the furniture of the living room like I was *NFLs* Hall of Fame running back Emmitt Smith, locking my fat ass in front of the television engorging myself to sleep.

I remained home for the next five and a half years focusing on my degree. Unfortunately, all those years after flunking in and out of college forced me to stay in school more than I wanted to, but I had to endure it, so I could finally get my life going as some kind of professional. Considering my tuition money went towards my education and fast-food joints, my bad eating habits included acting like *Nintendo's Ninja Gaiden* to feed my addiction. I broke the 400-pound zone for the first time in my life during this duration. I just hoped that it would be the last time.

# THE MODEST BUMP INTO

*I*T'S AMAZING WHAT TIME can do to lifelong crushes. During this time in my life, I pushed about 350-pounds, was unemployed and still living at home with my parents (redundant? Yes, but all too true.) I made an early decision to go to my local superstore past midnight to avoid any chance of any conflict of sorts all for the sake of not being seen. I had gone about a year without a "bump into," so I knew I was due for one, and that *moment* would be this day on a midnight trip on a Tuesday night where the odds were zero to none. Of course, that wouldn't be the case.

Initially, I was going to start a diet the day before on a Monday, but naturally, that never took. I spent that day wallowing in my own self-pity until the midnight hour where I committed to going on a midnight run to *Wal-Mart's* Superstore and buying nothing but rabbit food and kicking Tuesday's ass.

I perused through the organic produce section of the store contemplating to buy a box full of expensive ass organic carrots, or the *Wal-Mart* brand full of pesticides and poison for half the price. I weighed each in my palm like lady justice and leaned towards the *Monsanto* infused carrots all for the sake of saving a dollar. I tossed the bag in my cart, and when I turned, I saw my all-time high school crush, Mayra. Initially, we didn't make eye contact, but I noticed instantly that she had gained a tremendous amount of weight. I mean seriously, she must have been pushing 250 to 260-pounds standing at about 5'4. Her enormity infused me with such confidence, that instead of running for the hills so she wouldn't experience my enormity; I filled with confidence and tapped her on the shoulder eager to see a fellow counterpart.

"Mayra, is that you?" I asked.

She turns her complete body in a near "about face," and scans me quickly smiling.

"Oh, my gosh, Tre. Wow! How long has it been?" Mayra said elatedly.

Mayra leaped on me to give me a hug, as she kissed me on the cheek.

"So, how long has it been?" I asked.

"Since we graduated back in 99," Mayra said.

Mayra told me about her life, and in doing so, I was completely enthralled not by her interesting story that consisted of her and her three kids, but because I couldn't stop surveying her body. Considering I was also a fat fuck, for some strange reason I was so excited that I was naively on the other end for the first time. Strangely, I hoped that she was a nervous wreck talking to a man who at one time in high school fooled around with one another during a debate tournament when we were both freshmen in high school.

While keeping my smile and nodding in rhythm to the cadence of her story, I noticed the dark ring around the back of her neck replicating mine as a physical sign of sugar addiction, as well as her haggard exhausted look as spry hairs from her prominent bun laid sparse over her neck as if her neck was growing pubic hair.

For some strange reason, I was attracted to her. I knew behind all that weight was a woman who at one time was everyman's crush. Even her current smile gave a tremendous tell that she was once a stunning legend back in high school. I wanted to grab her by the hand and pull her in like that one fateful day freshman year when our debate teacher

Mr. Harmon paired us together to monitor the halls; eventually leading to a night of making out and heavy under the clothes petting; I rubbed the tip of my right middle finger a mere 15 years later and couldn't help but smile.

"What? Why are you smiling like that Tre? Mayra said smiling herself.

I wanted to tell her if she recalled that great day when we were just mischievous kids, but I knew she was way past that. Besides, why would she remember such a day?

"No, no, I'm just happy that you're happy," I said.

Considering Mayra was as beastly as me, my memory of her superseded any physical monstrosity that was being held by her worn exhausted attire; as was mine that I wanted to make love to her, and fully round the bases 15 years later, or at the very least instead of a stand-up triple, make it a fucking home run.

Mayra and I talked for another 15 minutes and eventually checked out together. We'd exchange numbers in which I would never call her but having her number a mere decade and a half later, and a couple hundred pounds later made me feel young again, and for the first time in years, I was the main attraction.

# HUMBLE-PIE: VOL. II

*W*HEN GETTING SERVED "HUMBLE-PIE," most people will learn from the experience and correct their mistake or whatever their calamity of bull-shit that occurred. Sadly, for most large people when they have a "bull-shit" humble- pie *moment*, unfortunately, because of what we've done to our body when it comes to skin elasticity, we either buy better fit clothes or simply lose the weight. Either that, or it's an uncomfortable situation; a task that is going to take months if not years to achieve. Deservingly so? Perhaps, but for other regular-sized people when they have a "humble-pie" incident, usually weight has nothing to do with it. For us large and in charge people, a "humble-pie" *moment* usually has to do with a "bump into" or "tearing" of the garment of sorts, or the all too common uncontrollable "misty inner body fragrance" or of course, the unnecessary amount of sweat that occurs in an air-controlled environment. Thankfully, this "humble-pie" *moment* dealt with the "uncontrollable sweat" in an A.C. location, so it was not as disgusting as the other options that I have certainly experienced.

\*\*\*

It was Christmas 2010. I was two-plus years into my solitude and certainly past 300- pounds again. A few months after I moved out of Tone's apartment I reached the 300-pound barrier, only to lose about

70-pounds in a four-month span. As much as I'd like to say that I kept it off and reached my usual goal of 180 to a 175-pounds, it seriously felt like the day I hit 231; I went back to 300 the next day as I've mentioned before. I would say in the next following year and a half I would balloon up to 300 by falling back into old habits and having to pull out my old solid black t-shirts again. To say I embraced the 231-pound life would not be accurate, although I did have two encounters with girls that should've validated my weight loss, but in all honesty, I fell off the wagon just as fast and as hard as I got on it, in that four-month time frame.

During this fall I wasn't a good brother, son, or tio. I fell back into my depression and made few family appearances predictably. The sheer emotion of pure disappointment from my meteoric fall was just too much to handle once again. Because of my absences from family functions, I knew I had to make it up to my family for never really being there on my deep downward slope, so I was desperate to make up any past grievances any way possible.

My nephew Zeke celebrated his birthday in September, and not only did I make a "hi and bye" appearance, but I didn't even give him a gift. Fucked-up? Absolutely. The reason I never bought him a gift was because I wasn't working at the time completely living off the residuals from my financial aid which let's face it went **ALL** towards "Fast-Food Alley." Another aspect was that my family has all their birthdays and occasions from May through September which my brother and I would dub "Murderer's Row." Naturally, buying gifts when you're unemployed certainly can be overwhelming especially when you're hitting the late months, and in this case, it was the finale of "Murderer's row" which was my nephew's birthday and I simply came up short which is why I bolted after the cake was handed out. Thankfully, my nephew had an abundance of gifts, so I knew my gift would have been lost if I ever gave him one in the first place. Not buying my nephew a gift naturally stayed with me throughout the months leading towards Christmas since I have a hard time of "letting shit go" which is petty, but to be honest although I knew my family could care less about gifts, I needed to do something of significance just so I could feel some kind of validity.

It was the day before Christmas Eve, and I had 13 dollars to my name. I wanted to buy Zeke a huge fire-truck loaded with toy cars which at the time he was INSANELY into. The problem was the fire-truck I did want to buy him was $39.99. I knew my dad would've floated me the extra cash, but I was done with those days of asking my parents for ANYTHING. It was bad enough after spending years on my own that I was back home. I then realized what I had to do. I had to pawn my computer and car stereo that I never took out of the package.

On the way to the pawn shop, I became infused with self-doubt and loathing all because I couldn't believe I was at that point. I was 29 years old, and here I was pawning my only two shitty assets. Thoughts of *When am I going to grow up?* Consumed me to the point of making my attempt in college seem trivial. I pulled up to the pawn shop.

It's always strange walking into a pawn shop because you know that you're about to give up something you earned, all for the sake of getting an ass whooping for a few measly dollars. Then there's the other feeling where you think that you'll get a good deal, and exit with the hopes, that "I'll be back to get my shit" which of course rarely happens.

I approached the counter with both car stereo box and laptop on hand, and I noticed the pawn shop employee looking at me already knowing how much to offer even before I placed my stuff on top his counter. After plugging in everything I owned to make sure it worked he'd asked:

"How much you want for the car stereo?"

I remembered I paid $200 for the stereo that had never been opened until now, and even though it was about a year old, it was in pristine shape.

"$200 man; it's never been used or opened," I said.

The pawn guy nods his head optimistically while inspecting my stereo. I was beginning to feel optimistic.

"I'll give you 35 dollars, and $50 for the laptop." He said.

A rush of endorphins flushed against my nerves as I could tell my brown skin was turning red.

"Hell no, are you crazy? That laptop is fast man, and the stereo is tip-top!" I said infuriated.

"Both your car stereo and laptop are outdated; that's the best I can offer you."

"Come on, I need the flow." I said desperately wanting to leap over the counter so I could sit on the motherfucker and rob his register."

"Sorry, I can't budge. Besides, I have a lot of laptops just sitting here, and to be honest I'm offering too much for your stereo that doesn't even have an auxiliary cord." He said.

I knew if I went anywhere else I'd probably get the same offer of 85 total dollars, so I knew I had to submit or go home, but I was desperate.

"Can you add $10, please man?" I said with my head hanging in defeat.

"No sir, I'll give you an extra $5, but that's the best I can do," he said.

"Okay."

My knuckles were fisted, and the Rock of Gibraltar had made its appearance again, and in deep frustration, I took the cash. I knew I could have thrown a fit, but in all honesty, I was defeated. I was already at the "bottom of the barrel." This *moment* here at this dive of a pawn shop only solidified that I was lower in the "bottom of the barrel" if possible.

I had a hundred and three dollars to my name. Not only could I buy

Zeke his gift but could buy him something extra all while having enough to eat *Whataburger* for the next few days. I couldn't wait.

***

Christmas Eve finally arrived. Normally, my family opened gifts now rather than Christmas day not because we were anxious for the presents, but because my relatives lived in Corpus Christi. We made it a ritual to open our gifts the day before in our home, so we could celebrate with us only, then on Christmas Day open our gifts with relatives. It was a ritual that I enjoy even to this day.

Growing up, we always spent our Christmas day with my tia D. She had a nice two-story home in a great suburban neighborhood. I especially enjoyed it because my older cousin Catherine had this kick-ass superhero action figure collection that was held on top wooden panels covering an entire wall in their personal action figure pose. My little brother and I would spend hours at a time gawking at her collection tempted to play with them, but because she had a strict "no touch" policy, we would sit and admire each action figure from a safe distance. Looking back, I would have to credit Catherine for teaching my brother and me how to appreciate, and respect other people's property, a lesson I hold dear to this day.

Now, most families with kids waited until midnight to open gifts, but because we were at my tia D's house, and Catherine was much older, they didn't mind opening gifts until sun-up. Needless to say, that my brother and I patience was tested. So, we would stay up as late as possible hoping that we'd get the call to open gifts much earlier but eventually would fall asleep on the floor together next to the action figures feeling secure knowing that they'd protect us from any kind of evil.

That morning my brother and I woke up to the clanking of pots and pans banging against one another that announced my tia and tio's aromatic breakfast. Considering I was excited about opening gifts, I was also as excited to devour my tia D's fluffy eggs and bodacious bacon strips– the combination of their breakfast, and gift opening was parallel to well... bacon, eggs, and opening presents.

Without brushing our teeth, my brother and I leaped from the floor and hurdled down the stairs three steps at a time. Halfway down from the stairs I stopped and from my vantage point, I saw my family and relatives huddled around the tree in complete glee as if they had been celebrating 30 minutes earlier. I noticed my tia D sitting on top of a bike. My brother slid into the gifts like Ricky Henderson back in his prime. For me, as I slowly went down the stairs, I couldn't wait to see why my tia was sitting on top such a cool bike. Now, this bike was no ordinary bike. It wasn't one of those old people 10-speeds, or those corny ass mountain bikes (which I currently own,) but it was a BMX bike. *What?* I thought. It didn't make any sense as to why my tia D was on top of a BMX. Tia D would go on a tangent saying things like. "I can't wait to start using this bike to exercise or go run errands with it to "la Esquina." Before I could think of how she would be mismanaging the bike, my mom hands me a box about a foot in length and a few inches in height. Now, my family at this time could only afford one gift per person, so I was never expecting a multitude of presents, so I knew what my mom was handing me was pretty much it. On a few occasions, she would also give me a small thoughtful gift to express how much she loved me, but that was really all I ever expected, and to be quite honest I was grateful for that.

I shredded through the wrapper in an instant, and what it was would be a staple in my attire pretty much until today. It was the all-white *Nike Air Force Ones.* I'm not sure how she knew I wanted those shoes, because I never spoke a word about it once, and let's be honest even if I said the brand, I didn't think she ever knew what to look for. The only way I can see that she may have known was because of my addiction to the TV show "*Yo! MTV Raps.*" I was always talking about the shoes my favorite rap artist sported, and maybe the one time she saw me gawking at the *Air Force Ones* just registered to her.

I leaped on my mom giving her a kiss on both cheeks followed by a big hug telling her "thank you!" Suddenly the bike wasn't shit until my dad tapped me on the shoulder with my tia D holding the bike like it was ready to ride.

"Sonny, this is also for you." With my *Air Force Ones* in my hand, my jaw dropped to the crevasses of the Earth's core; I was in complete shock. I leaped onto my dad and his little sister, Tia D and simply said "thank you" *numerous times.* Everyone from my sister, brother, tio and cousin Catherine were silent in observation as their smiles expanded further than the Corpus Christi Harbor Bridge. I inspected every detail of the bike from its solid black frame to the black tri-wheel rims and gray tires– it was glorious, and most importantly it was perfect. I placed my pointer finger on the red striping on the side of the main frame and streaked down the entire bike in complete admiration. I couldn't help but think how my parents could afford two kick-ass gifts. I also thought, *when could I ride it?* I couldn't wait to go home and have it all to myself and begin a career as a BMXer at the young age of 13.

After admiring perfection, I turned to my parents, and while my mom held my little brother and my sister rested her head on my dad's shoulder admiring my sheer glee from a distance, I'd ask my parents.

"Why both the *Air-Force Ones*, and the bike? I asked bewildered mostly because we were a family of little means.

"Why not?" Mom asked.

And that was it. Her response is exactly what I should've expected from her, and I couldn't have been more grateful. I knew when I asked both my dad and mom about the gifts I looked and processed what "greatness" truly was for the first time outside of my sports heroes—I was finally growing up, and as much as I'd love to say that *moment* became a substantial point in my life, I was maturing. Looking back, I wished I knew of my parent's hardships, and what they did to overcome them back in the days so maybe they could feel that we knew of their greatness and sacrifice then. Considering that I come from great humble parents, I knew that they never searched for praise and would have never wanted to put such a burden on us because they worked hard for their children and wanted to give us the childhood they never had or could've ever expected to give, and I thank them for it.

It's in this memory that I've always wanted to be what my parents are. Which is why pawning what I "needed" for the sake of giving my nephew a great gift was always worth it especially if I received only a smile and a hug. Although I knew Zeke would've never cared if I had a gift to give or not, I suppose I just wanted him to look at me the same way I looked at my parents that Christmas Day—which he always has. Unfortunately, in the cross-hairs of my wonderful plan to exceed those Christmas expectations, my addiction superseded my original intent.

***

Predictably, I used a portion of my pawn money on food on top of food, on top of food. By the end of the day, I had $25 to my name. So out of the one-hundred and three dollars going directly to buy Zeke his gift, instead, I hit two restaurants and was $12 richer than when I went into that pawn shop. In panic mode, I went to the toy store in search of a "smaller "version of what I originally wanted to buy him, and thankfully I found a shittier version for $19.99. Instead of a large fire truck with about 5 toy cars, there was a blue wrecker with two toy cars included.

It wasn't what I originally wanted to buy Zeke, but it would have to do.

Christmas Eve was here, and I must admit I was a bit nervous, but after seeing my nephew open his gift, and immediately rush to me to give me a squeeze (which was our way of saying a hug) it nearly made me faint with tears as I held back desperately despite my goose-bumps reflecting a Vietnamese minefield. I couldn't help but think *why did I have to buy that shit food? the firetruck would have lifted him to the moon.* I lifted up Zeke as high as I could and gave him the biggest "squeeze" possible followed by numerous kisses as he pulled himself down so he could play with the blue wrecker.

I can't help but admire his youth realizing that I could've given him anything, and he would've loved it, much less just being here would have been enough. As my nephew played with my toy all while in the box, and neglecting the others, the wattage coming from my smile was enough to light the darkest cave, as I was never so relieved, and finally happy, as happy as that day my parents gave me those *Air Force Ones* and the BMX bike.

I saw that Zeke was having trouble getting the wrecker out of the box.

"You need help mijo?" I asked.

Zeke would hand me his toy. I sat back in my sister's chair near her kitchen table and untied the knots and do-hickeys that were keeping the wrecker attached to the box. I could see why my nephew was having such trouble.

*Jesus Fuck!* I thought.

I realized the only way I could get this damn toy out of the box was by getting scissors and a Phillips-head screwdriver. Zeke looked and waited in anticipation as I was ready to toss this toy across my sister's living room out of frustration. I did my best to unhinge this thing, so I could see Zeke embrace it fully. In the process of getting this toy out of the box, I began to sweat profusely, considering it was 32 degrees outside. Instead of being buttoned up in a jacket or hefty sweater, I was wearing my trusty old black t-shirt with red gym shorts.

A bead of sweat plunged to the top wheel of my nephew's toy. I wiped my brow, and the back of my hand was as glossy as a freshly waxed *Maserati*. I asked Zeke for a glass of water, as he rushed to get it like he knew I was dying of breath even though I was sitting down on a lovely padded chair. After Zeke handed me the water that I inhaled in one swoop, I then felt a sharp pain on the side of my right rib– it was a cramp. My right hand quickly comforted my side nearly causing me to drop the wrecker. I squinted in pain and tried not to alert my family who was in the living room enjoying the early morning. I would've hated to alarm them of my pain on such a wonderful day. I asked Zeke to give me a paper napkin so I could wipe the sweat, but most importantly so he wouldn't see me in pain.

Frustrated, I took a few breaths and the searing pain faded. I attended to the toy. After wiping my face and neck sweat, I finally released the wrecker and handed it to Zeke as he began to play with it on top of the tile floor. While trying to recover from my discomfort, I was in too much pain to see Zeke embrace my gift fully. I eventually regained my breath and was somewhat 100% free of pain from that side cramp I just endured. By this time my nephew had been called by my sister to give him the other gifts. I stared at the abandoned wrecker and glanced at Zeke as he embraced his new toy. I smiled gratefully that he had such joy.

I waited about three minutes to rush to the restroom to make it appear that I was somewhat okay from opening Zeke's gift. I lunged over the sink taking in as many deep breaths as possible. I looked into the mirror. My long hair which at the time was to my shoulders was soaked with sweat. My black shirt had a large ring of sweat soaking the neckline about six-inches down, and my face was red as fuck. I swear I resembled an NBA star getting ready to play his fourth overtime. I took a seat on the toilet and rested.

Forty-five minutes would pass when someone knocked on the door.

"I'll be right out; the ham got me good!" I shouted out loud confused as to why I would shout-out such a thing.

"You want to play with my toys tio T?" It was Zeke; I quickly get up from the toilet embarrassed.

After I jolted from the toilet, I look into the mirror. Thankfully, I wasn't red anymore, but my shirt was somewhat still moist from my sweat, the ring around my collar had dried providing a white ring.

*Fuck!*

I turned my shirt inside out, and thankfully the white ring wasn't there, but the neckline was stretched. I stared at the mirror after I splashed my face with cold water and took a breath of disappointment. *You pathetic bastard.* I said to my reflection.

I went to my nephew's room, and he was giving all the love to the wrecker, and I couldn't help but smile realizing with great pain comes great love.

# TRUE LIES

$\mathcal{G}$ROWING UP, I NEVER had a problem with weight. I may have been a chunky kid from time to time, but through my junior high/high school years, I was a pretty good athlete. I was always in the park playing football, baseball, or basketball since I was good at those things. Okay, maybe I was above average at most playing basketball. So, when I say I can't pinpoint an exact moment I fell off the wagon, it's no lie. As much as I'd love to say I developed bad habits with exes, I knew it was an amalgamation of everything that led me to gain all my weight. To blame others is just a lie I tell myself to keep me sane.

Many of the habits that are common amongst obese people are, wearing the same clothes, becoming reclusive, growing the clichéd beard, or having long hair to try to cover-up the unfortunate self-inflicted flaws someone of a large physique endures. Probably the most damaging flaw common amongst my fellow obese people are the lies we tell to avoid not only "bump intos," "judgments," or "risk" being in an all "booth" restaurant– which I'll explain later. This is why we lie. Most who have become reclusive will gain an additional 10-pounds whenever an impromptu hang-out with friends occurs. Unbeknownst to those friends who simply want to hang-out to catch-up, they will never know the inconvenience and pressure we endure knowing that your sincere offer to hang-out is met with haste and self-deprecation in preparation just to spend an hour with an old friend.

These thoughts normally begin with predictions of every step I'll take to ensure that one: we don't have the "dude, you're gaining weight" talk, and two: how to avoid an accident or embarrassing moment. Such examples are: will I fit into their car? Am I going to burst into a cold sweat for simply walking from the car parking lot to the entrance of a building? I mean how embarrassing will that be if I'm out of breath from walking 30-feet. Another example would be: "Do I have to order a light meal, so I don't prove those staring at the large man right?" These are some thoughts that run through my head before even committing to chill with my homeboys. Now, I know that these are "self-inflicted" wounds, and doubts that I deserved, but to be honest, I'll come up with some clever lie to get out of an occasion while thinking, I'll make-it-up to my homeboy in three months when I'll lose even more weight since we last hung-out; which at the time would be a good six months later. *Will I ever lose the weight?* Of course not, if anything I'll weep and reflect on my glory days from when I was in shape and lived a decent life all while spending the night eating Buffalo wings stacked higher than my 5'11 frame.

Because of these lies, I've lost friends and family. It got so bad that I've canceled great moments from friends and relatives because of these tired out lies all ranging from graduations, weddings, funerals, and life achievements. Instead of attending such moments, I'd rather lie and stay home clogging up my arteries. "The Recluse life choice" has certainly taken precedent over risking a night of discomfort to experience such occasions with great friends and family leading to not only losing touch with them, but moving on from them, as I'm sure they have with me, and deservingly so. As much as I'd love to say that I love them all more than the entire Universe would be false because even though they are second to my life, I've chosen the all mighty burger as a far greater friend that I do my friends or family. Selfish? Damn- right! But there is something that ignites my taste buds when I just think of food, and although exhausting the glee I receive with every bite is simply everything to me while releasing me from any stress or loathing I may have from canceling on family, and friends.

Jesus fuck! I had great friends, and I just pissed them away. Now, I live this sorry existence, and as much as I'd love to say that "I'll make-it-up to them" as I'm completing this sentence, I'm eating a burger and climbing two proverbial Everest's to one day weigh a 180-pounds, so I could make-it-up to everyone. But that seems to be a longer hike every day. Unless God claims me early, for which I deserve; we will all reunite soon in which I'll certainly make-it-up to them then– I promise.

***

My best friend growing-up was Walter Gutierrez also known as "Disney" – obvious reason. We were from the same neighborhood, went to kindergarten together and were close our entire lives— best friends to the fullest. Our whole thing growing-up was going to the movies, concerts, and reciting as many In *Living Color* and Chris Farley quotes as possible.

Our first movie together was *Powder* and the many concerts we went to spanned from *Alice In Chains, Metallica, Scorpions, Bone Thugs N Harmony, God Smack,* and many others. *Blue Oyster Cult* was our first concert; Jesus fuck! we had a great time hanging-out almost every day. We were on such great terms that we both were on "walk-in" bases at each other's parents' home. I even recall, in a lame attempt of dropping out of high school for almost two weeks, Disney letting me crash at his crib during school hours for every one of those days. I mean we both truly looked out for one another, and I can honestly say we had love for each other in everything we did.

After high school, Disney and I floated from job to job doing nothing with our lives. By the age of 25, we had already flunked out of college twice, were roommates once before, and had worked about ten different jobs. One day while staying up late chillin in my backyard just "shooting the shit," we both decided to go for a walk around my neighborhood to smoke-out. It was a sweet innocent time that we were trying to harden ourselves by becoming amateur chain smokers. Earlier that day we went to the movies and watched *Sideways*. That movie was so inspirational to us that we spent that entire night talking about how great it was. From the triumphant return of Thomas Haden Church who is a Rio Grande Valley native, but what captivated us from the movie was the writing. Disney and I always believed that we were the pseudo-intellectuals of movie reviews this side of the world, certainly in McAllen, Texas.

On that long walk, Disney and I discussed what we wanted to do with our lives. The majority of our conversations leading up to this point normally concluded with Disney becoming a head manager at the many local telemarketing companies that he and I occupied throughout the years, and for me, I always assumed that I'd take over my pop's finance business which almost happened.

As our walk continued, we eventually came around to "Let's get into the movie business. What do we have to lose?" For Disney, he would want to become the next Tarantino, while I desired to be the next great screenwriter especially after watching the film *Sideways*. As we turned the corner of the alley towards my home, we were inspired. We were so inspired that we pulled an "all-nighter" strategizing how this dream was to come true.

Eventually, Disney and I created a few scripts, won some local film festivals, and eventually worked for a big-time "low budget" movie in the Austin/New Braunfels area. When we both came home from that film, we were set to make the next move and do whatever it took to one day become Hollywood dynamos. Eventually we'd be contracted to work on other people's local film projects leading us to become pretty good in our craft.

About two years into trying to bust into the film industry we both grew frustrated with the constant struggle, as finding pay for being a production assistant (P.A.) had become exhausting. The closest I ever came to do anything substantial was working on a *PBS* Show called *History Detectives* as a P.A. Eventually, my dad asked me to join him at *Finance Capital*, and the rest was history.

When I worked for my father, I went in weighing 282-pounds, and when I lost over a 100- pounds, I gained half of it back by the time Superman lost his cape. I also moved in with Tone and learned about the "recluse" life, and completely fell off the wagon… again.

As for Disney, he kept hoping to bust through and get to Hollywood. He eventually found his own crew all while asking me countless times to join him in his new filming endeavors. Of course, I repeatedly declined with my many "made-up" lies. I knew he knew I was lying, not because he knew me for decades, but he knew it wasn't likely for me to ever pass-up writing for a film, especially together. I gave him the excuses such as: "I'm working late tonight" to "I have to go to a closing for my dad." At times these statements were true but were mostly a lame attempt to make me sound busier than I was. The main thing that was sincerely bothering me was that I was lying to the GREATEST best friend anyone could ever have, all for the sake of vanity for which I knew Disney would have never judged me in the first place.

One day, I received a call from Disney telling me that he completed his first film with his "newly" acquired crew, and he was going to have a premier two-months later. I was the first person he called. Until that phone call, I hadn't seen or hung-out with Disney for about three months. By this time the longest I had ever gone without seeing Disney was about a weekend, so three months was unprecedented. Disney asked:

"So, what's up brah? Are you going to make it?"

I thought within a two-month time, I could lose 25-30 pounds and be back to my old weight.

"Hell yeah dawg, of course, I'll be there."

"We're going to also have a wrap-up party tonight downtown; you have to come," Disney asked.

I squinted when my infinite "*Rolodex* of lies" shuffled at lightning speed desperately searching for an excuse to get out of tonight.

"Damn dawg, I'm leaving town this weekend to close a deal, but we'll hook-up for sure when I get back on Monday," I said.

I nearly punched my office wall as I was full of rage and disappointment. I knew I was letting Disney down. His greatest achievement and I knew I should've been there, especially because of what he meant to me.

"It's all good man; be safe on the road and we'll hook-up later dawg," Disney said.

I spent the week devouring value meals, and extra ketchup packets pissed the fuck off knowing damn well that I wasn't going to lose enough weight for Disney's premiere that was two months away. I then passed the 250-pound barrier, and for the next eight years to a decade our relationship was never the same. We saw each other sporadically, and yes, he saw me at my all-time worst at 401-pounds. Considering how close he was to my family, he never met my nieces and nephew either. Also, the achievements that he and I obtained in that near decade we'd both be absent from; all while his absence was justifiable.

I always imagined Disney and I having one last real moment together with "Blackbird" playing in the background for some strange reason and forgetting about the last ten years without one another and picking up where we left off. I know it may be wishful thinking, but one day I'll throw my "Hail Mary" pass, and we'll be close again. But, if he decides not to attempt to catch my lofty pass than I'd most certainly understand, but in all sincerity, I hope Disney gets all he deserves and more. I just hope I'm there to see him get to his ascension.

Disney made a splash in the R.G.V. market as a local film legend and even had a few films make it to *Netflix* and local *Wal-Marts*. It always made me smile every time I would see a copy while perusing for a 5XL t-shirt. As of today, he moved on from filmmaking, and became a family man with a gorgeous daughter.

If I could ever sit Disney down and apologize, I would say: *Sorry for leaving you stranded for personal vanity, and although I know you would've understood and never judged my struggles, I'll do everything I can to rebirth our legacy together.* Knowing the great guy Disney is, he'd make me apologize to everyone else I had left stranded in this silly self-sabotage that I could never thank him enough. For Disney, I miss you and love you brotha— "Wish you were here." An inside joke from our Pink Floyd phase.

> *"Can* **WE** *order your 50-nugget special with large fries and*
> *a large soda?" I asked*
> *"Yes, did you want to add our New York cheesecake for an*
> *additional $2.50?" the drive-thru attendant asked.*
> *"Yes,* **WE** *would like to add that please," I requested.*

# GOOD TIMES, BAD TIMES

$\mathcal{S}$OMETHING HAPPENED AFTER I lost all my weight the first time from when I weighed 180- pounds at the age of 26. For most people when they lose a dramatic amount of weight, they either get into a long-term relationship and quickly gain their weight back or stay trim and go balls deep into the bachelor's life and expose it for what it was— a period of time filled with clichéd sex and debauchery. For me, because I had a deep regret of never experiencing the "college life," I did everything I could to fill that void when I lost 100 plus pounds the first time around and exploited my late 20s for everything my "college life" should've been which included women, having many "Joe jobs," and of course getting arrested again and again.

When I had my rebirth at the age of 26 life seemed easier, expressive, and most importantly fun. You would've thought that I would have fought to stay in shape, so I could enjoy the fruits of my labor of running eight-plus miles a day just so I could fit into a medium shirt with room to spare and finally have my neck back. I suppose those weren't in my cards, or as a man of faith would say: "maybe God wants me to endure a 220-pound explosion so when I get back to weigh less than 180-pounds, I'd learn my lesson, and enjoy life once again."

Now, during this time, I was 26-years old working with my pops at *Finance Capital,* living on my own with Olivia. My life consisted of

8 a.m.-5 p.m. work, and to be honest because my pops was the boss, I usually strolled in an hour or so late which was immature, but when I got there, I was ready to work and always gave a 100%. So, from 9ish to 4:45ish I put on a daily performance of a lifetime enjoying working with my father until those last few months when I saw Superman lose his battle with Doomsday.

From 5:30 to 6:30 I ran and became a "beast" to the fullest. I mean I had a killer stride just crushing those miles. After my run, and clean-up, I went out to a bar, and nearly got trashed every day, which to be honest since after Lauren and I broke-up at the age of 21, drinking was at an abundance. I never drank at home, because that's where I drew the line. In a way, it was my way of telling myself I was not a drunk or alcoholic. When I went to my local spot and drank myself to a sludge of domestic shit beer, the night would conclude with me either hooking-up with some "random" or having a friend drive me home or to their place.

Those following mornings naturally led to an awkward drive to pick-up my car at the bar, as I'd either be asleep the entire way or at the very least have one eye squinted open to harness any bright sun-beams while silence overwhelmed the car ride to not add any more pressure to my hangover.

When I lost weight, this happened quite often, and because of the dramatic weight loss, it was easier to get trashed. It was also easier to pick-up whichever girl I wanted, and unfortunately, put up a lame performance in the sack, or as I like to frame it a "self-absorbed" performance. To be honest, at the time, I didn't give two fucks.

Besides the constant alcohol binges and numerous "random" liaisons, I was also arrested twice. They weren't alcohol related, but I caused trouble and did not take care of my responsibilities, leading to traffic warrants which I would eventually get busted for. Unfortunately, the first time I was arrested led to an awkward but unsurprisingly confrontation with my father the man I refer to as "Superman."

***

When my father closed the doors to *Finance Capital,* I knew my livelihood was about to change. I had about a year and a half of good times. By the time we closed, I had lost my way from a 180-pounds and running 8 plus miles a day, to weighing 256-pounds and sitting on my ass 18 of the 24 hours. The toughest part of my day was using my time for embellished gluttony and far and in between sexual encounters.

I still didn't adhere to being a drunk by any means, but at this time in my life, because I was at home, and had a decent savings account and no rent to pay, I could feed myself with fast food and cheap beer. I still wasn't bringing the beer home, but the little savings that I did have was going to stale beer and the hot bartender that I never had a chance to ever close, especially as a renewed fat-ass. Predictably, every time the hot bartender was there, I'd say to myself "if I had never fucked-up, I'd be getting these drinks for free, all for the price of a "me-centric" love-making session." All that I could settle for was giving her a large tip, so I could at least see a smile pointed my way— sometimes it was about the little victories.

While living with my parents, besides being on the "bottom of the barrel" I was on a complete decline. I was approaching my late 20s; 250 plus pounds soon turned into 300, then 350, and eventually a whopping 401-pounds all while being unemployed. At least I was still going to school by the time I reached my all-time heaviest. Now, I know there were bigger crises going on in the world, but I was going through my predicaments, and at this point, I was spinning out of control causing some kind of vortex in the bottom of the barrel, and there was no way of getting out.

Before "reclusivity" became embedded into a decade-long lifestyle; my public parameters were the shitty bar and Mom and Dad's house. When I would go home, I would only use it for the five "S's" "Shit, Shower, Shave," and the occasional deluxe sandwich and multiple sodas all because I couldn't afford my famed "deuce" from *Whataburger*. Thankfully, *McDonalds* had a shitty dollar menu, which in retrospect I'm sure I would've chopped some heads looking for chump change to find a dollar to eat the $1 double cheeseburger from *McDonalds* saving my life.

\*\*\*

In this process, I endured my first arrest. One night, my homeboys Luis, Disney, and I decided to hit up a strip joint where it was B.Y.O.B. So, of course, we bought two cases of brews. On the way, we ended up getting pulled over. I recall pulling over immediately, and as the cop approached my window asking for my license, without even thinking if I had any warrants to my name, I was more concerned that my homeboy Luis had an open beverage in the car, as he hid it well besides his boot. I trusted he wouldn't do anything stupid hoping this would be a routine stop and prayed that I'd only get a warning. Instead, the cop asked: "Sir, can you step out of your car?" Luckily, I lived in an area where it was mostly populated with Mexican Americans, so I didn't have to worry about getting smoked for being brown and proud.

"Fuck!" I shouted in the car.

I handed the keys to Disney who was in the passenger seat.

"Take my keys in case they take me in, and whatever you do don't call my pops," I said.

I tried to be cool about the process, as I didn't want to provoke fear in Disney and Luis, but I knew when I told them "not to call my pops" it be a dead giveaway that I was about to shit myself. I slowly stepped out of my car, as the cop stepped up to me looking me dead in the eye trying to intimidate me.

"Do you know why I pulled you over?" The cop said pissed.

"No sir? What's the problem?" I said trying to stay composed.

"You have a warrant out for your arrest. Now, turn around so I can cuff you."

"Wait! What! I'm not aware of any warrant officer!" I pleaded to the cop.

"You can figure it out at the station."

I saw Luis and Disney looking at me with a combination of "What the fuck!" to "What an idiot." Of course, the cock-sucking pig put the cuffs on so fucking tight, as he threw my newly fat ass in the back seat nearly breaking my arm. I mean I was in serious discomfort and pain.

"Yo man, can you loosen the cuffs, please? Jesus fuck!"

"What was that? Jesus what?"

I guess he was offended by my use of Jesus in what was a desperate plea. I mean I thought at the time, and even now that my use of Jesus was appropriately used. My wrists were pinched, but my elbow felt so tender from him pushing me into the car. I was arrested in McAllen, but my warrant was from Edinburg our neighboring city. He drove me to the corner of what was a boundary between Edinburg and McAllen. Now, no one was there to begin with, and I started to think *"Oh shit! Is he going to beat the shit out of me, and leave me for the crows handcuffed?"* I tried getting answers from him, but he was just an asshole cop and ignored me which made me consider that maybe he didn't get laid that morning, or perhaps caught his chic with a dude who most likely resembled the

180-pound version of me— in that case, I didn't blame him.

Finally, another cop car came, and before we switched handcuffs, I asked the new guy if he could loosen the cuffs, and thankfully he was cool with it, as the McAllen cop looked at me and the Edinburg cop like we were both pussies. The drive to the Edinburg police department was filled with conversation, and even while he booked me, we had a delightful discussion on how he thought petty warrant arrests like mine were not necessary. The cop also made it clear that if it were up to him, he never would've arrested me; he said: "There are serious crimes out there, and here I am booking you for some dumbass misdemeanor unpaid ticket shit." Of course, I agreed. We also discussed how he passed up his dream of starting a custom car shop, but because of an unexpected leap into fatherhood, he had to find a gig with great benefits.

After I was forced into the closest cell near where I was booked, I stood proud against the bars in my socks. Thankfully, he kept me company, and instead of talking on my part I just sat back and listened, not wanting to ruffle any feathers to where he could make my life even more miserable if he wanted. What I considered "bad-times" because I never wanted to get arrested in the first place; ended with a good conversation as he ended with "maybe one day I'll open that shop," all while looking at a picture of his young son in his wallet.

Now, I know this wasn't hard time, but my 30s were fast approaching, and I was on my version of the "bottom of the barrel," and now arrested sitting in a jail cell. What made things worse that night, was without realizing my homeboys were all poor fucks, so I should've known while sitting with the Edinburg cop that there was no way they were ever going to bail me out. I asked the cop "What if I don't get bailed out tonight?"

"Well, you won't be able to get out until you see a judge Monday morning," the cop said.

I began to wonder how jail food tasted, and maybe this was a blessing in disguise, and I could drop a few pounds looking good for the judge Monday morning. This thought predictably rambled through my mind as a first-time offender. The officer eventually left me to myself, where I spent the next few hours reliving my past from my glorious high school years where I was a popular dumb-ass slacker, to strangely my two major relationships with both Lauren and Ana. I also reflected on the many random one-night flings I had throughout my 20s and eventually that one and a half year of bliss where I fit into medium t-shirts, and size 31 jeans. I also remembered how bad-ass it was to rock a stylish solid shirt with fitted jeans while rocking *Air-Force Ones or white* "shell-toe *Adidas*" with a black on black Yankee cap. *Jesus Fuck! I was a bad boy.* Now, I know for a fact that I would've indeed had tossed the McAllen cop's wife back in the days, which would've made him tightening my cuffs justifiable.

I smile knowing how silly I was with those insane thoughts; when surprisingly the officer came in, unlocking the jail cell.

"You're free to go," he said sounding just like the movies.

"Seriously?" I said.

"You must have great friends."

"Oh shit." I thought.

I waited to sign out. I remembered Disney, and Luis had just gotten paid, so maybe they were able to pull their money together and bail me out—that would be sweet. The only problem was *How the fuck am I going to pay them back?*

I finished signing out, and as I exited the door, there were my homeboys, as they reached for me for a group hug.

"I can't believe I'm hugging a felon," Disney joked.

"Very funny my man, but I'm all good."

"Damn bro, it was a scene out of Cops when they arrested your ass," My homeboy Luis said as we all laughed along.

I looked over Luis towering frame as my chin rested on his shoulder, and saw my pops standing like a large statue with somewhat of an emotionless expression. I'm sure it was more of an emotionless expression of embarrassment as he looked at his oldest boy coming out of jail and joking with his homeboys as if nothing happened. I was positive this wasn't his proudest moment.

I looked over at the clock, and it read 3:17 a.m. If my pops was upset, maybe it had to do more with him being awake so early rather than seeing me out of jail. I slowly walked over to my pops.

"Sorry, Dad." I wanted to burst into tears as I hung my head in sheer disappointment looking for some comfort.

"Let's go home son."

On the way home, I expected nothing but silence and deep sighs of disappointment rivaling when he would see me walk-in with fast food bags an hour after our family dinner. His ability to guilt you without saying a single word could crack a steel wall.

To my surprise, my dad was cool as shit. Not only was the ride to drop off Disney and Luis easy, but the drive home was comprised of my dad's childish humor consisting of *Looney Tune* whistles and being an upbeat person that he has always been blending well for a great night that camouflaged my shitty night.

After we dropped off everyone, my pops and I stayed parked outside our driveway and talked. No scolding or discussion about how much I disappointed him occurred. We just chatted about his life as a man, and how important Abuelito was, and how much we both missed him. It was a therapy that I didn't know I ever needed, but yet sincerely felt was necessary for me to have that night. We continued to talk leaning against the back of the truck for the remainder of the night until the sun crept up, turning the dark sky into a smokey blue. As the peppered flickering starlight's dwindled, it was my first great night as a man. When Dad and I were about to conclude our conversation, I asked one last question that until this *moment* was never a concern or even a thought, but I suddenly had to know.

"Why aren't we a family that hugs or tells one another that we love each other?" I could tell I struck a chord to my father's great heart.

"You know I love you and our family more than anything in the world, right?" My dad asked.

"Of course Dad, I've just always wanted to know why we weren't one of those types of families."

"To be honest, I wasn't raised that way either. Always being there for one another was good enough. Especially the neighborhood you and I grew up in. The person who grew up with a father in the house was considered "rich," and "lucky" in those neighborhoods. Also, your mom and her sisters your tias had to grow up fast because of their father's drinking and second preferred family. Her father made your mom hard, and I suppose without realizing that we didn't have to wear our emotion on our sleeve. If I could change anything, it would certainly be us being closer, because I need it too. I'm so sorry about that Sonny."

"No need to be sorry Dad. You know I love you very much, and to be honest after Abuelito died, I saw something in you I had never seen before," I said.

I could tell Dad was curious while restraining his tears. Dad tended to get emotional whenever Abuelito was mentioned.

"Which is?" Dad said.

"That day at Abuelito's funeral. For the first time in my life, I saw that your hardened exterior had been taken from you." I said.

"Losing Dad was something I thought growing-up would never happen and seeing him there at his rosary only made my biggest fear real."

"I know Dad. I can't imagine that either."

I reached in for a hug and clasped onto my father with a grip that could never be unhinged.

"I love you Dad."

"I love you too Sonny."

The last time I hugged my dad and told him I loved him was at my Abuelito's funeral.

# THE WORST DAY OF MY LIFE

*F*OR MOST PEOPLE, "THE worst day" in someone's life usually consists of a tragic accident, a lost loved one, bankruptcy or foreclosure amongst many other things. For me, and for those close to me, my worst *moment* was when I was in a car accident. I got t-boned by a drunk text messaging cocksucka driving 60 mph into my then precious 2003 red *Chevy Impala* nearly sending me to an early grave to hang-out with my beloved Abuelito and dog "Casper the G.O.A.T." for which I'll explain in a later chapter. Another worst day for me was when the doctor told me my liver was four times larger than normal, which predictably was met with a fried food combo of sorts. Another was when I was told that I wasn't going to graduate high school on time and seeing my mother's expression of disappointment was all I couldn't handle. Then there was being bailed out of jail by my father. All these examples fall in line as my worst moments, but sadly fail in comparison as to what I've always considered "The worst day of my life."

I recall the exact date that it occurred because "IT" was a day that I never thought I would ever experience which was: May 10, 2014, also known as the "day I graduated college." The fact that I graduated considering what kind of student I was in public school for most would consider getting their diploma their greatest day. As for me, it was anything but.

Now, how could this day be known as "the worst day of my life?"

Well, as of May 10, 2014, I weighed exactly 401-pounds. Before that fateful day in May, I hadn't weighed myself for a few months, but I knew I had reached new heights of lateral expansion. My bad-habits combined with the stress of completing a final semester did not help. It was predictable that that spring seemed to only consist of late-night papers with nightly glutton fests mixed in with a habitat of "slothery, and solitude."

Now, the only reason I weighed myself the day of graduation was that I went in with the idea that this would be the day I begin a "new" journey. As a new college grad (history) why not use graduation day as a starting point to once again one day weigh within 180 pounds. Did this stick? Of course not, but it was a nice idea.

***

Two weeks prior, I went to the University's bookstore to measure for my cap and gown. My cap came in at 7 5/8, and my gown was labeled "infinite plus." I know that isn't an actual size, but I knew the lady was thinking it, and let's be honest I was the perfect model for an "infinite plus" size if there ever was one. Although the gown resembled the tarp for a baseball infield, I was just grateful that I had something of size. I mean how embarrassing would it be to show up in my greased-stained black t-shirt all for the sake of not fitting into a fucking glorified solid black muumuu. Thankfully, the gown fits with change. Of course, I wouldn't touch it until graduation day.

Now, this day meant more to my parents, because out of all my siblings the odds of me doing something with my life seemed improbable. I mean there was a time in my life where the idea of becoming a manager to a retail store was my ceiling.

***

As we approached the parking lot of the convention center the day of my graduation, I couldn't wait to see how people reacted to the logo I put on top my cap, which for many graduates had phrases such as "College Grad," "Class of 2014," "I'm Available for Hire!" or my favorite and sadly too true "$40,000 Dream Come True." For me, I wasn't having any of it. I figured since I knew I looked like Shamu on a bloated day that I had to put something on top of my cap that summed me up in one phrase or image. I thought back to when school was a struggle for me, and I vividly recalled my friends always thinking of me as some "hip-hop historian," and here 15 years later hip-hop was still the main source of my identity… besides my obesity. None, of this so-called "mumble rap, hip-(p)op, or my favorite gentrified rap." But I always stuck to the old school, and sure as my then expansive CD/tape collection consisted of paramount figures such as Big, Tribe, Nas, Eric B and Rakim or my then favorite Eazy E. I knew I had to do something that would identify with hip-hop, so I decided to go with the group that many had always recognized me with, and that was the Wu-Tang Clan. I remembered I had the yellow Wu-Tang logo decal with the "Wu-Tang" written in the center of the Wu symbol. That day of my graduation, I grabbed the cap and carefully placed the yellow decal on top. It looked so fresh and so clean that I even tweeted the photo of the cap to RZA's twitter account. Although I never received a repost of the image, I had never been so proud to represent the Wu in my finest day as a human.

After we parked at the convention center, I put on my gown which thankfully fit nice and loose. I took a few photos with my family. Normally, I would've preferred to take those photos in the privacy of my parents' home especially because it was a cool 105 degrees outside, and I surely resembled a beached killer whale. But I was here, and I knew the goal for the day was to receive my diploma, and not roll an ankle upon crossing the stage, and risk the stage collapsing forcing the ceremony to close all because the night before I had gobbled down an entire large meat lovers' pizza and liter of *Dr. Pepper.*

Everything went well until they lined us up to take our walk. By this time, I was sweating and sitting in between two dime pieces. I tried to joke with them to give them the idea that "maybe if he was in good shape, I'd certainly sleep with him." As I was of course thinking: *If I was in good shape, we would've slept together to relax our nerves in the green room before crossing the stage.* The ceremony commenced, and without a hitch in the plan, I crossed the stage without rolling my ankle, and because I concentrated too much on that possibility, I didn't take my time to embrace everything I had overcome to finally earn a degree that I thought I would never achieve in my life. I mean seriously, my first job out of high school 15 years earlier I was separating chilies in a subzero fridge, and now here I was earning my bachelor's degree. Instead of jumping to the sky in celebration my thought was seriously not to roll my ankle or fall which was more of a possibility because I didn't have the ability to jump anymore anyways.

After the ceremony, I took a few more pictures with my family holding my papered diploma sincerely happy that I didn't tumble on stage. I mean seriously folks, not falling was on my mind the entire time.

After taking 9 million photos, I suddenly received a barrage of *Facebook* hits saying "Congrats." Confused, I checked my phone, and my brother God bless him, posted pictures of me, and to be honest, what I saw suddenly turned a cold sweat that had been obtained in that cold ass convention center to a heated onslaught of perspiration glistening and enhancing my rosy cheeks as it rivaled the red from the *UFW* flag. My heart fluttered as I broke into an insane sweat. *What the fuck?* I thought.

My brother posted at least 10 various photos of us, but the first pic was the only one that I had to look at as rage overwhelmed me while I tried to keep cool just so I could appear in a good mood for the sake of both my mom and dad.

I looked again at the photo, and I had never been so disappointed in my life. I couldn't believe how HUGE I looked. The only thing I could compare it to was when my mom called me a disappointment after I told her I wasn't going to graduate high school on time— talk about coming full circle.

We decided to have dinner at *Red Robin* my then favorite burger joint. On the way to *Red Robin*, instead of commencing in a conversation about my big day, as both my mom, dad, and brother had many various questions, I would respond in rushed contrite answers all while deleting my brother's post and figuring out how to configure my *Facebook* page so that none of my exes would see me at my ALL-TIME worst. I checked the messages (all were from old friends) including a friend of mine who said the first day of high school many years earlier that always stuck with me that "I'll probably drop-out and amount to nothing, and probably die by 25." In retrospect, this almost happened. Her comment was; "I'm super proud of you old neighbor." So, that was a small victory.

I finally configured my *Facebook* the way I wanted it; where no one can "tag" me in a photo without my permission. The only problem was that my brother had about 30 friends that we shared, so whether I'd liked it or not, that photo was going to be seen, and I'd be forced to take the loss. I could only pray that none of my exes or random's didn't see shit; just the thought of it now is horrifying.

I knew a good 45 minutes had passed from figuring out how to configure my *Facebook*. While eating and responding to questions in "yes, no, uh-huh, and yup" thoughts swirled about those damn pictures as I began resenting my little brother Jesse who was sitting across from me. I understood that Jesse meant no harm and that he was proud of me, but he had to know I looked like shit in the picture? Right? I've stated before that I was never the greatest brother to him, perhaps this was his great revenge for all the bull-shit I put him through. Which in that case all I have to say is "Bravo!" and well deserved.

I wouldn't receive any more notifications about my obesely photo. I knew my ex Ana had been friends with my brother, and maybe had seen the picture which would have devastated me. I could only imagine her gawking at the photo thinking "I loved that man? He's fucking huge, GROSS." Or perhaps she didn't see the photo, which I'll probably never know, and to be honest I don't want to know. Either or, taking this defeat on what was supposed to be my "greatest day" my day of redemption from when I was supposed to be dead at the age of 25, instead turned into a self-conscious, vanity-filled day.

My mom currently has my graduation photo from *Facebook* hung-up on her living room wall for everyone to see. When I visit my family, I make a conscious effort to avoid eye contact at all costs. Perhaps when I get my masters and eventual doctrine, I can proudly replace that *Facebook* photo with a picture that will be known as my "Greatest Day of All Time."

*"Yes sir, can I order your Blue-Ribbon burger, with endless fries?" I asked.*
*"Of course, is there anything else you want?"*

A few relatives and family friends had joined us at *Red Robin*, and although I knew I could order the left side of the menu, I didn't want to become a spectacle.

*"No, that will be all."*

# IT'S IN THE DETAILS

*T*HIS IS PROBABLY THE toughest chapter I've written. I must admit that every chapter until this one has had its variances of difficulty, but this one is the toughest because it's the most revealing. When I thought of this book, I told myself that it had to reveal the physical stresses of an obese man, whether that be my day-to-day addictions, or the often-overlooked reflections of what I used to be before I fell into this whirlwind of gluttony, or at the very least what I did to get back into shape. Unfortunately, I'm still an entire Everest from achieving my goal. Of course, the person reading this book may find it as a book of "wallowing, and self-pity," and that's okay because, in all honesty, these moments that I have been writing about is for those who not only want to understand the duress that we obese people endure, but it's also for those who are in a similar situation so they could know that they are not alone in what is most likely the most stressful enduring time in their life.

I'll begin with a question every reader has on their mind which is: "Does your penis become an innie?" The answer is once you reach a certain weight unless you're a "pipes-man" of sorts, then, unfortunately, various forms of "innies" do occur, and that's because the pelvic area (sorry for lack of scientific terms) contains as much fat thus most likely inhaling your penis. As for me, I have enough slack to where I didn't become a complete "innie," but I will admit that at a certain weight you see your body change to the point where your body becomes completely unrecognizable. As for what happened to me, my pelvic area ballooned up incredible inches. My thighs resembled sacks of potato's infested with dimples that the jiggle they contained along with my hanging gut caused a calamity of chaos around my once vibrant "pleasure zone." This led me to ask every time I looked in the mirror *What the fuck!* This is why I grew to ignore mirrors. With the enhancement of my thighs and the surrounding areas, it deemed an optical illusion of what was once a proud member of my body.

Another question that many people have asked me is: "Does your sex drive diminish?" Now, I've talked to other 5XLers, and some have none to minimal problems in the bedroom. I don't know; maybe they were bull-shitting me; after all, this is a sensitive subject, so I can't blame them. As for me, and as difficult as it is to admit, I certainly was affected. I mean before I fell off the wagon onto a landscape of yellow wrappers and 32-ounce sodas, my sex drive was admired by even the greatest Adonis's— which is what I like to tell myself. Getting women back in the days was never a problem for me until I discovered the loveable "deuce" from *Whataburger.* I'll say, by the time I hit 330-pounds I simply lost interest in approaching women. For Christ sakes, just getting "hard" was tough to get. There was no way I would've had confidence even if at 330-pounds, I was somehow able to pull off a miracle and have a girl want to sleep with me. It just wasn't worth the possible embarrassment upon engagement if possible. By not wanting to look at a mirror any-more, and simply being tired to lug around an additional 250-pounds with me every second of the fucking day, it made it impossible to lead a happy sexual life, much less life itself. Just completing these sentences is embarrassing, and maybe something I need to endure especially with the idea of my family reading this, and now having them look upon me with all speculation becoming confirmed by this chapter. I could only hope that it'll never be a topic of conversation. I can imagine my mother pulling-out the neck and giblets from the turkey on Thanksgiving Day feeling sorry that her oldest son can't relate. Then again, maybe I could tell them to skip this chapter altogether.

If awkwardness from my family happens, then I'm okay with it. If my jokes about my obesity offends anyone, then they need to understand that humor often gets us through another day especially when a fellow obese man or woman drown themselves in a pile of burgers and are most likely on the brink of a physical/ mental melt-down. After all, we would never want anyone we know or love to ever experience what we are enduring. Besides other obese people, there is no one else to understand our problem unless they have been obese themselves or suffer from any other kind of heinous addictions.

So far, I've listed two physical changes that are beyond embarrassing. Another struggle I've endured that is common among the obese is simply keeping maintenance. As much as I'd like to say it's an "additional 5 minutes" in the shower, it's more like 20 minutes. Now for women, I can imagine they'd enjoy more time because most women love showers, but for men, the majority want to get the hell out and start their day. Believe me; I'm certainly one of those men.

Now, for most obese men we know that the odds of us ever finding love after surpassing the 300-pound barrier is sincerely 5 million to 1 (exaggeration.) Often times we default to the same attire, and sadly hygiene takes a back seat. Besides, the 300-pound lifestyle is a huge contributing factor to being alone.

For me personally, while I rock the same black t-shirts that remain in heavy rotation, I admit that I do take pride in two major things when it comes to hygiene, which is one: my hair, and two: my teeth.

I'm thankful for being blessed with a phenomenal head of hair, and a decent smile, so brushing is essential for both aspects especially when finding balance out of my obesity.

A majority of those years of discomfort came during my college days from when I weighed 401-pounds. Despite walking across campus, you would've thought I had lost crazy weight, but that was not the case. Actually, a four-year plateau ensued as I used my financial aid money not only on overpriced books but also on the insane delicious tacos that were straight across the university or "fast-food alley." So, it was easy to beat the fuck out of an order at this taco joint after a day of school as my attention went towards Mexican history and their greatest culinary contribution— the taco.

By the time my day ended, I had reeked of sweat and straight-up funk as embarrassing as that may sound. With the unhealthy combo of sweat and gorged skin, it was easy to lose yourself in a day of perspiration making you rush home and take a shower to get rid of the funk.

Now, I must admit there were many days when I got home and said "fuck-it," and instead of hitting the showers I'd simply engorge myself in *Burger King* all while my funk would dry-up; as disgusting as that may sound, it was very much true. I mean seriously, I knew my days would consist of school and food, whether that was me eating at the *Burger King*, or eating it at home. Unfortunately, food became everything to me, even when a hot waitress served me. I knew that there was no way that she would find me attractive, so why not spend the night filling my hole thinking that I would've certainly had banged any waitress back in the days.

When you become 400-pounds, you acquire new funk. However, I'm still a germaphobe even to the point where I've washed my hands so many times that I've gained rashes between the webbing of my thumb and index finger. You would've thought I'd take care of myself even better, and as I've mentioned before, I'm not even sure how I got this far.

So, back to the showers. I needed an additional 20 minutes just so I could gain some kind of freshness, and come out of the shower believing that I was somewhat a 100 percent cleansed. But what was almost certain, was that I'd come out that shower out of breath sweating profusely with a side cramp like I had just pulled a muscle, all because of the strain I'd put on myself in the shower. Unfortunately, the freshness would last less than a minute. From the time of brushing my teeth to my 10-foot walk to bed, I'd lay down to sleep drenched in sweat and some deep panting. It was seriously that bad.

Now there are remedies to stop the sweating besides not moving at all which is *Gold Bond* Powder that people use to put on their undercarriage. As for me, I tried it once, and never used it again mostly because it grew cakey. At the time I was walking across the university constantly, and that powder would compile into a goop of funk. I would tell myself "you know what I'll just shower twice a day instead… as one should." This of course rarely happened, but because it was truly painful to stand longer than 10 minutes showering twice daily became impossible, as I'd like to attribute it simply to not having the muscle tone to stand for two 30-minute shower sessions especially after an entire day of walking across the campus.

Another aspect that was certainly a surprise to me was fucking skin tags. I mean seriously, what the fuck was that? What the fuck is it? As if my ever growing bulbous 13-gallon *Hefty* sack of belly wasn't enough. Now I had to endure these skin flake protuberances that resembled a miniature(s) brown elephant ears. For me, they were mostly located in the arm-pit area. They didn't hurt or anything, but they were certainly a visual disturbance causing me to ignore my underarms and my undercarriage. I

mean it was hard to look at a cluster fuck of skin tags considering I had
many more physical issues that I was dealing with. On the other hand, I
still had my hair which thankfully God had blessed me with, and in all
sincerity is the only thing I have going for me... physically. Then again,
it is beginning to gray, but who knows that could be a good thing.

As if skin tags weren't enough, the next onslaught of physical blem-
ishes was a form of skin tag or sty occurring on my eyelids. Although they
weren't as large as what masqueraded under my arms, they were these
specs of pimple like bulges resembling any high school girl's worst fear on
prom, but instead of being on the nose they were on my fucking eyelids.

At the time I received a cluster of pimples on my eyelids. I had just
lost my job, so I had no insurance to get them checked out. I attributed
it to being a fat fuck and theorized that whenever I decide to lose weight
that the eyelid skin tags would naturally disappear. Of course, I also
looked to the Internet for answers. Most of the message boards said that
they were related to high blood pressure, but in reality, all the photos
that I saw from my research resembled nothing like I had. I mean for
Christ sakes they were miniature specs at best which was something I
would've killed for, and instead, I had a barrage of zits on my eyelids
for which I had no answer.

Because I wasn't working at the time, I didn't have to be seen by
anyone and be forced to answer the question; "What the fuck is wrong
with your eyelids brah? You look like Chris Elliot from the movie *Something About Mary.*" Such a question would've made me laugh, and at the
very least I could've responded and said something to the effect of "I was
born like this dude," and snarl the fuck out of the cocksucka.

As the years passed, they did somewhat go away because I constantly
picked at them. They scarred, leaving me with very few eyelashes from
when they were long and lush before. At least with scarring, they left me

somewhat approachable. Poor Mom, I could only imagine her looking at my eyes from across a restaurant table wondering what was happening to her once magnificent son, and probably thinking my last days of life were coming sooner rather than later. Seeing that in her eyes, it wouldn't much matter because I'd still hit that *Whataburger* "deuce love" like a mother fucker later that night.

After about a year of trying to weather the storm of sties on my eye-lids, I woke-up Christmas Eve with a new sty on my eyelid, and it was not just another ordinary sty; instead it was a rather large black sty on the bottom of my right-eye-lid appearing like a large mole that would've made Cindy Crawford's mole look like a damn freckle. *WHAT THE FUCK!* I thought. Thankfully, I just started my teaching career and was able to acquire decent insurance and getting paid just enough for a single guy to thrive in a town of about 6,000 people. I instantly set-up an appointment with a dermatologist and wouldn't see him for another two-weeks.

At the time, I worked an hour away from my hometown and came home to visit family and friends for Christmas. Now, because I couldn't get this mole off my eyelid until after Christmas break, I couldn't see my old homeboys whom I hadn't seen in months. I promised them and myself that I would visit especially now that I was losing weight at the time— well sort of. My family ignored my obvious newly acquired friend, and when I'd go back to school my students would also ignore my "black target"— they're so sweet. You would've thought junior high kids would've called me out.

Finally, I was able to get an appointment with the skin doctor, and Jesus fuck the procedure was painful. First of all, when he asked me to lay down on that uncomfortable leather recliner with that meat wrapping paper, I imagined I resembled a beached whale especially when the doctor walked in, and his eyes bulged with hunger; possibly assuming that I was going to be a "long-term" patient seeing nothing but dollar signs because of my health. Thankfully, I had insurance.

The cocksucka approached me, and I was grateful for the shower I had taken earlier, so the risk of smelling like a sweaty 70s snatch wouldn't create a clouded divide as the doctor approached my speckled eyelids.

The doctor pulled out an aggressive looking syringe.

"Jesus fuck! Are you kidding me Doc?

"Close your eyes; it's going to sting a lot, and whatever you do DON'T MOVE. AFTER ALL, I HAVE A NEEDLE NEXT TO YOUR EYE.

I was suddenly hit with vertigo and could sense the needle approaching my eye as my body mended with the recliner. I felt the needle pierce into my black sty, and it felt exactly how I thought it would feel and sound. It was as if someone was piercing a well-done turkey with a thermometer breaking the crackling skin sounding like a popped tire. As my eyes jetted with tears, my eyes remained pinched shut as the doc continued with my other three sties. While the doc pierced into me again and again, he mentioned that he had never seen a sty like the first and would take it in for a biopsy. Of course, hearing the term BIOPSY overwhelmed any pain I felt from the shots. Suddenly, I heard the pinging from the syringes being placed on some sort of metal plate. After he was done poking through my sties my senses flourished, and my eyelids remained pinched.

"Now listen; those shots were for numbing. Now, I'm going to cut off a few of your rather large sties with a scalpel. It's not going to hurt, but it is going to be uncomfortable."

I would feel him slicing away at my sties feeling like a rusted shovel grazing a pebbled concrete path.

*Holy shit what the fuck!* I shouted in my head as I wanted to leap out of this chair and beat the fuck out of this guy.

"Please lay still. I have a scalpel next to your eye."

After the final slice, the cocksucka was done.

"Go ahead and lay there as long as you want and hold this over your eye."

It was a napkin. I only laid on top the recliner for a minute desperately wanting to get the fuck out of this shit box. I opened my tender eye, and there were literal holes in my eyelids. I held the napkin over my eye as the napkin resembled a teen's spotted rag.

The drive home all I could think of was: *Dude; I can have cancer.* Now, I have a rather old car, so there was no auxiliary cord to plug in my phone to listen to some jams, or podcasts as I drove back to my new home. It didn't matter anyway because the only thing playing over my head was the doc saying, "I've never seen that on an eyelid before, it MAYBE CANCER." Okay, I may have added that last part, but he may have well just said that anyways.

I wouldn't get my results until two weeks later when I waited in the examination room for over an hour only to hear the nurse pop her head into the room and say, "You're okay, thank you." A one hour wait for a three-second reveal. I should've been pissed, but I was ecstatic about the results, and couldn't wait to go home to take a much-needed nap which had voided me for those two weeks.

I had many more physical alterations within these bulbous years of mine such as stretch marks that resembled a Jackson Pollack painting of skillful bedlam if it ever existed. I also had a magnificent pair of "man boobs" that any flat girl or woman would desire. After a while, my body resembled everything I hated.

"Can I have 3-foot-long chili cheese dogs with a large order
of chili cheese fries, and a 64-ounce grape slush? I asked.
"Is there anything else you want for your order?"
"**We'll** also take a corn dog, please. And please don't forget
the mustard." I asked.

# III
..

# THE MIND
*of a junky*

# I'M BIGGER THAN AN NFL OFFENSIVE LINEMAN

*E*VERYBODY WHO KNOWS ME understands that my passion and knowledge for sports is limitless, especially football. If I had to list all my favorite sports teams it be the: *Dallas Cowboys* (of course), *San Antonio Spurs, Mexico Futbol, New York Yankees*, and of course my beloved *Texas Longhorns* for which I hold Jeff Fisher solely responsible for killing the career of the greatest Longhorn of all; Vince Young, but I digress.

I recall one evening watching my Cowboys play on a Sunday night with my entire family. I always made it a point that no matter what I was doing that I'd always watch the boys with my family. By this time in my life, I weighed a whopping 331-pounds. Why so specific? Because that Friday, I had an appointment with a doctor about my liver (results were stunningly bad) so coming to my parents' home to watch the game was a great relief of stress. That was until Jon Gruden began talking about the massive offensive line from my Cowboys. Gruden stated how large the left tackle was by being 6'5 325-pounds. My first response was *Jesus fuck that's a big boy.* Then like a linebacker blindsiding a quarterback, it hit me. *I weigh more than that motherfucker?* I would end up putting myself through a torturous inner monologue of various bits of how I was such a disappointment such as; I *outweigh this guy by six-pounds, and I'm six inches shorter. At least he looks good in his uniform.* That left tackle was the greatest version of 325-pounds I'd ever seen. There was also the obligatory: *imagine how I'd look in a Cowboy uniform at 5'11 331-pounds? I'd probably resemble those poor dogs that are dressed like humans and are forced to stand on their hind legs.* The difference was those offensive linemen that weigh 325-pounds and are 6'5 are physical freaks of nature, while I fall along the lines of being a 330-pound, 5'11 freak of gluttonous nature.

# THE SPECTACLE

$\mathcal{S}$OMETHING HAPPENS TO THE psyche of men and women who hit the 300 to 400 plus pound range. We see for the first time the slight eyes of others. For example, when we enter a building most will ignore, but most if not all will express this shy form of gawking. It may last a split second or seconds, but as we read everything your glance says, and believe me when I say this; an eagle's squawk would be drowned to a silent murmur when it comes to the eyes of those who have a fucking staring problem. Variations of "Jesus Christ that's a fat fuck," or "Poor guy, that's a big dude," or "Gross, he has bigger titties than my girl does," or "Wow! That's unfortunate; I'll pray for him." Whichever of those thoughts is used just about sums up the gist of whatever your eyes are yelling. It's the obese equivalency of seeing a homeless person on the street and walking past them with "spectacle eyes" saying "bum should get a fucking job," while never knowing their personal situation.

What I'm trying to get at is that your eyes tell your thoughts, and we can read them like Shakespeare. This, when of course we are at our all-time low, because although we want to fight our addiction; unlike drug and alcohol addicts who can avoid temptation by simply avoiding a bar (easier said than done of course,) for the obese and the entire Earth, we must eat. Now we understand that we can order a salad with water from the menu designed with bright colors and the infinite additives they put in their food just to keep people like me ALWAYS coming back like the cliché of a weak addict. In doing so, I'll use every excuse for my downfall, and in this case not being able to say no as I walk into a fast food establishment.

After seeing all the eyes of disappointment or disgust, we try to walk with blinders, but your stares and the occasional "look back" as we pass one another beams right through our blinders like Superman's laser eyes, leading us to walk up to the counter and whisper our order in hopes that you don't hear and confirm your speculation of us.

***

Normally, I wake-up starving, and instead of just getting up to go pick-up something to eat, unfortunately, I strategize where to go where the odds of a "bump into" is less likely. Now, I know what you're thinking "if this guy put as much energy of where to go into eating less, he'd get back into shape in no time," and you're right. Now, on this particular day, I wanted one of those old-fashioned breakfasts rather than picking up a drive-thru order, so I decided to go to this local Mexican restaurant joint that's pretty out in the open, and besides it was 7 a.m. and more than likely I'd be the only young person there apart from the old souls where the odds of a "bump into" would be less likely.

I beat the sun to the Mexican restaurant, and surprising to me there is a small but substantial line of older peeps— old men of course. I walked towards the end of the line, and instead of hiding eyes of judgment, I received long gazes and agape jaws wide enough to consume my desired over-the-top breakfast in one fell swoop. Strangely, I respected them for their blunt facial expressions because of me being a spectacle.

The door opened and upon entering the restaurant the first thing I noticed besides the hot waitress which I knew if I was back in my prime,

I could've picked her up and been forced to leave a larger tip, but I digress. Besides the hot waitress, I noticed the booths. Pissed, I grew frustrated because it was a "booth only" restaurant. Now, for most people booths are great because of their extreme comfort, but when you weigh 401-pounds, often times or at least for me, unless the table of the booth isn't entirely bolted to the floor, the odds are, that I'm not going to fit, or at the very least be insanely pinched. So, for future sake, those of you who go to a restaurant with a rather large exceptional person, please choose a table instead of a booth. Believe me; we already know that we are a physical spectacle; there is no reason to put us in physical pain as well.

Normally, I could instantly tell just by looking at a booth if they were "big-man certified," or if I was about to endure 30-45 minutes of discomfort, and in this case, it was certainly going to be uncomfortable. I sat down and sucked in my gut, so I could appear thinner to the waitress as much as possible.

*Damn it!* I screamed in my head.

"Will this do?" The waitress asked sitting me to my booth.

"Sure," I said in searing discomfort.

Because of my years as an obese beast, I've learned nearly any possible "worst-case scenario" to help me out of such situations— especially the one I was currently in. As I was annunciating the word "sure," my mind was shuffling through a *Rolodex* database of how to get out of this shitty "worst-case scenario," and that's when it hit me.

"Sure," I said.

I rose from the booth as the waitress looked at me askew, and I asked.

"Can you grab me an Arnold Palmer while I go wash my hands?" I asked.

"Arnold Palmer, no problem." She said.

"Thank you."

I smiled and took a lap to the restroom while really looking for a damn chair.

*How the fuck can a restaurant, have all booths and no chairs?* I thought.

I couldn't help but think as I rinsed my face over the restroom sink. *The owner must be some fat shaming cocksucka who knows that when he designed this shit restaurant that one day a fat fuck would need a fucking chair.* I ran my hair under the faucet and exhaled in disappointment.

After I exited the restroom, I saw the Arnold Palmer occupy my booth from a distance. While walking across the restaurant, I noticed one of the old men ogling his eyes at me and nod in sheer disappointment, as if his thoughts were "That's why we're the fattest nation." I shyly grimaced at the old man's presumed thoughts and thought: *If I was sure that my ankle wouldn't roll-over, I would sack that piece of shit and bust his other hip.*

I squeezed into the booth and turned back noticing the dime-piece counting her till, and because I was pinched, I went from a 58-inch waist to a solid 50 making for a painful but welcoming feeling.

At this point, I knew what I wanted to eat, but these old guys kept staring at my direction. Finally, I waved one down and said sternly across the restaurant. "My man, can I help you? Jesus fuck!" The old man turned away as the hot waitress comes to take my order.

Now, because the waitress was a certified dime piece, I knew I was in a delicate situation. I knew if I ordered a meal I really wanted to have, then she was going to look at me for the spectacle that I am except with a pinched gut. On the other hand, if I ordered a low-key meal, I could salvage some respect from not only the waitress but also deny what the old geriatrics would expect of me to order.

I looked at the waitress's caramel eyes and told her my request. I could feel the deep anticipation from everyone in the restaurant including the dime-piece waitress preemptively placing her thumb under her order sheet just in case she needed another page to complete my order.

"*Okay… I'll order your large breakfast with an extra egg and cheese. Can you also include a stack of pancakes?* (The "large breakfast" originally included: 3 eggs, 2 sausages, 3 slices of bacon, a side of refried beans with tortillas.) The dime-piece wrote on her notepad like an ambitious journalist writing in shorthand.

"*Okay, will that be the 3 or 5-stack?*"

I looked over towards the geriatrics and could sense that a few of them won some off-setting bets.

"*The 5-stack please.*"

While burrowing away in her notepad, I noticed her eyes swell with disgust.

"*Um… is that it?*" she asked.

I smirked at her tone. I tried to lean back in disappointment but obviously wasn't able to physically do so.

"*Just a refill,*" I said defeated.

"*Okay, that'll be the large breakfast with an extra egg, and cheese, and a 5-stack of pancakes?*"

"*Yes.*"

"*Okay, it'll be right out.*" She said impressed with a slight hint of "Oh my God!"

# FINDING MECCA

*A*s I MENTIONED BEFORE, when I look back I can't really specify a single moment as to when I completely fell off the wagon. But I can attest to a "holy-shit!" moment that solidified my monstrosity of an appetite or addiction. For me, this day was the first time I shopped at the "*Big and Tall* store." As much as I'd like to say I weighed 401-pounds, but at least I was 6'5, instead I was barely 5'11 so that would mean that I was at the *Big and Tall* store not because of my height, but because of my weight, which this day would correspond with "THE WORST DAY OF MY LIFE" as it was my graduation day, or at least a few weeks prior.

I had to buy a long-sleeved shirt and slacks for my long-awaited event, and for the past three-plus years, I'd been rocking the same two solid black t-shirts in rotation with the same two gym shorts. Honestly, at the time I wasn't aware we even had a *Big and Tall* store, but in a strange way, the idea that I was in that realm of oversized clothing, I was somewhat relieved that I didn't have to go through the constant humiliation of just wondering if a department store had my size and risked having another episode like I did at *Wal-Mart* that near-fatal night.

I pulled up to the parking lot completely feeling defeated. Considering they had a wonderful display of mannequins dressed in nice clothing suited for the 32inch waist challenged, I was offended. I mean how could they have the balls to promote stylish attire for the morbidly obese? I understand that we should also have options, but really promoting the idea that "hey, you can look dope as shit if you rock a 58inch pant, and a 6XL button-down shirt" was complete bullshit! in my opinion. Now, I know I may be coming off as insensitive especially because I'm a big-ass man myself. But my aspiration is to one day rock reasonably sized attire rather than be outfitted into super plus sized clothing and reason with myself that it's okay to be large because there is now a store that carries outfits I can fit my spherical body into. Now, is wearing the two stained black t-shirts any better? Of course not, but I knew when I put them on, I couldn't stand being in them. The idea of finding great clothes to appease my shit physique could only compromise or prolong my desire to one day wear a suit without worrying if I look like a well-suited engorged tick.

I get out of the car. Now let me remind you I was at my heaviest at this point weighing well over 400-pounds, so getting out of a car wasn't as easy as I'd like it to be, but rather it took a nearly full body heave just to be able to step out. Yes, I was out of breath just doing so while also hearing my spine crackle and pop as I lunged out.

I approached the *Big and Tall* store, with a limp as opposed to the famed Tony Manero strut from *Saturday Night Fever* all while avoiding the reflective windows. When I stepped into its nice cool environment, I realized that I stepped into the Mecca, a Mecca rivaling Rucker Park in Harlem or the actual fucking Mecca for those with an over-eating disorder. I walked in and strangely enough, there were no "spectacle" eyes, no judgment, or no gawking– I was with my people and I was not the biggest person there.

As I perused the aisle, I saw sizes I've never known existed such as XLT, XXLT, and XXXLT and so on. The XL I understood, but what the fuck did the "T" stand for? I asked the girl behind the counter, and since she was a fellow "plus sizer" I felt comfortable to ask. I was feeling so good if I was a different person I certainly would've picked her up.

"Ma'am, what does the "T" stand for in "XLT?"

"Yes sir, it stands for 'tall,' so the shirts are lengthier."

"Okay, thank you," I said as my eyes swelled with optimism.

*Holy shit! The days of praying for a shirt to cover my belly were officially over.* I thought. Now, if I wanted to shoot basketball jumpers, or raise my hand to answer a trivial question, those options would be possible now. I wouldn't have to worry about exposing my gut or ass crack because the shirt would go well past my belly which meant there would be no more stretching my shirts after a wash. I was elated. I walked through the store with a smile on my face that extended further than a symphony of egotist–I was in heaven. I went through every rack picking clothes I never had the intention of ever wearing or buying. I just wanted to feel how it felt to fit into something for the first time in close to a half-decade certainly retracting my previous statement about the nicely dressed mannequins in the storefront window.

*Thank you, Lord!* I whispered as the mound of clothes in my dressing room resembled the rolling prairie hills of Texas.

Hours must've past, and I settled for a solid dark blue button-down sleeve 6XLT, and a 58-inch black slack with a belt as long as the aisle I was suited to walk in a few days for my graduation. Unfortunately, the 6XLT was their largest size, and thankfully it fit me well enough so I could sit down without risking the buttons bursting the seams. I couldn't wait to celebrate with a "deuce love" from *Whataburger*.

My euphoria wore off only to be replaced with grief as it would hit me that not only was I shopping at the *Big and Tall* store but that I actually enjoyed it, not to mention I only fit into their largest size. Sadly, the *Big and Tall* store became my home for years eventually having me resent those mannequins again, and permanently. To say I was in heaven would be an understatement because although I knew that this store would put an end to my black t-shirt collection, I knew it would only prolong my current obese physicality for years to come.

# HUMBLE PIE: VOL. III

$\mathcal{B}$Y NOW I'VE HAD my share of "humble pie," but as much as I'd love to flip the switch and simply say *I'll never eat fast food again*. Instead, I've had to deal with 10-pound monthly increments whether that is for weight gain or weight loss. A "bump into" or a "humble pie" experience is always at risk and sometimes it can be a more than one occurrence.

I had recently reconnected with my old buddies I hadn't hung out with since high school. We once had a "bump into" when I weight about 180-pounds after my first weight loss phase from when I weighed 282-pounds back in my mid-twenties. The next time we hooked up, I was passing by 290-pounds, so yes, I had gained 110-pounds since our first get together about 2 years before. Their "spectacle eyes" were in full effect considering that these guys were also not in the greatest of shape.

We had been hanging out for the past two weeks when we decided to go out to a fancy restaurant and take the wives along. Of course, I was the single one along with a single gay friend of mine who like me also had weight problems, but strangely was a huge endorser in wearing snug clothing. I'd love to say I admire his courage, but for me personally, I need to be cozy and prefer a stretched out black t-shirt sadly.

We all decided to go to a fancy Cajun seafood restaurant. Everyone was dressed nicely while I was of course dressed in my finer grease stained attire. Except for this time, I was able to bench my blue gym shorts for some khaki cargo shorts. Was I still underdressed? Of course, but it was all I had before I made the crossover to the *Big and Tall* store years later.

The night went as followed. While everyone including myself had dishes filled with the entire ocean of fried fish all while kissing their loved ones, my gay friend Jonas and I baked under a lamp that was directly over our heads like we were the ones getting fried. I mean while we both tried to act cool, and keep in dialogue with everyone else, both Jonas and I were perspiring like we just completed a marathon without the heavy panting. Instead, our shirts were drenched while beads of sweat turned into streams of perspiration. There was a moment when I was talking to Jonas about our "sweat" session when actual sweat sprayed off my top lip as if I had just gotten punched by Drago in *Rocky* 4. Jonas looked at me with "spectacle eyes" all while empathetically sympathizing with me because he was enduring the same discomfort.

By the conclusion of the night the sweat had created a Saturn sized ring around my t-shirt collar, and because I was constantly tugging at my drenched heavy collar throughout the night, my t-shirt resembled a 70s style V-neck except without that 70s bush chest hair. For Jonas, although his shirt was soaked, and dripping with sweat off the bottom tail of his shirt, at least he was wearing a dark flannel button-up camouflaging any wear on his collar– lucky bastard.

After we said our awkward goodbyes, I sat in my car and cranked the A/C for about 10 minutes cursing at myself continuously. That night on the way home I picked-up a *Whataburger* deuce and a bob breakfast, and it was great.

# HUMBLE PIE: VOL. IV

*W*HEN IT HAPPENED A fourth time, I couldn't call it a freak occurrence anymore. By this time, it was a trend or a way of life. I suppose after five-plus years of being voluntarily large that I was going to have my fair share of "bump intos," or "humble pies," and by now I was living on the edge with my ears perked as I waited for the next "humble pie" experience to occur.

This time in my life I was about five years into my large(ness) weighing about 330-pounds. I worked with my sister Karina at the time. Yes, that meant I'd worked with my pops, and now with my sister who had her own occupational therapy facility. She had her business a full year when she asked me to join her and be a filing manager of sorts. To me it was work. I had recently transferred to my local University, and it was the perfect gig. I was able to go to school and have some loose hours at work. The problem was that there was this insane unicorn of a dime piece working there. Now, until then I always took pride in having the ability to pick-up or talk to any girl no matter what level of hotness they were on. The only problem now was that I'd been 5 years out of the game, and I weighed on the lesser side of a beached walrus without the mustache.

She went by the name of Mia. What made her the all elusive unicorn was not only her spectacular smile radiant enough to emphasize the glow of the sun, but her affection in attitude was everything every man, woman, or child would ever look into someone. She was phenomenal. Her patience with children was inspiring, and her upbeat personality made working there an event rather than work. I swear when she would walk near my proximity, I could hear the Beatles song "Come Together," blast in my head as I'd envision my old self simply winking at her and having her fall directly into my arms as we'd fully engage.

Now, she had a boyfriend, but he treated her like shit, which if she was by any chance a walrus lover I could guarantee I would've treated her like the human living angel that she was. Now, I didn't really have the courage to talk to her all that much because I had been out of the game for years, and being out that long can mess with a person much less an obese person. As a matter of fact, about two months working with my sister I was barely able to pass by her and commence in cheap talk about our affinity towards the Spurs, and our Cowboys. Of course, I had continuous, predictable thoughts such as *if she had seen me in my prime we would've been together.* And since obesity was the hand I was playing; I was losing.

So, after six months of lame ass conversation with Mia, I was about 15-pounds heavier which I was convinced if she was single than I would've been 30-pounds lighter– ah who am I kidding? I was lucky to have been 15-pounds rather than 30-pounds heavier which was possible and had been done numerous times.

One day my beautiful sister walked into my workspace wanting to have an office diet challenge, and because Mia was pristine to the fullest, my sister put her in charge of the weekly weigh-ins. Ten people took part in this 3-month contest, so there was a chance that I could win a cool "G" which would've been perfect for my annual spring-break birthday. I was in, and to be honest, for the first time I wasn't wrecking myself into a cliched self-destructive whirlwind of shame as I approached the weigh-in.

The day of the first official weigh-in was similar to when I weighed myself that first day of school in swimming class. I purposely stood at the end of the line. The idea that my co-worker opponents were standing around the scale along with my sister and Mia didn't suit me. I certainly didn't want to provide the spectacle performance before lunchtime. I could only imagine what their conversations would've been if I could have been a fly on the wall after the weigh-in.

Finally, it was my turn, and Mia looking all types of "unicornish" awaited me as she held her Dallas Cowboys clipboard in her all black scrubs with pink *Nike* shoes. *Jesus fuck! she's sexy. Even her solid tone scrubs were no match for her bodacious curves.* I thought.

I was next in line, and suddenly I was drenched in glisten and nerves. I kicked off my new fresh white shell-toe *Adidas*, and luckily, I had a new pair of *Hanes* lite black ankle socks, not that I have funky smelly feet which is uncommon for an obese man, but funk or body funk I've always had control over- at least I'd like to think. Mia called me to weigh in.

"Alright buddy, you're next," Mia said.

I smile and instantly noticed the scale was one of those modern all-digital glass pane scales that had a maximum weight of 350-pounds.

*Oh shit*, I thought.

It was a *Moment* of truth. I knew that scale was about to be pushed as close to 350 as possible especially since I knew I was at least 345-pounds. *What happens if I weigh more than 350?* I thought. If the scale cracked or displayed some kind of error, I'd kill myself. Actual thoughts of suicide flashed in my mind along with a "deuce" from *Whataburger* as a final meal. I simply prayed that I wasn't past 350-pounds which at this time would've been the largest I've ever weighed.

I stepped onto the scale and as predicted everyone stopped what they were doing to see the "spectacle" adhere to the masses' assumptions.

Similar to "Humble Pie Vol: I" where I weighed myself in front of the entire class of youths and dime pieces, I awaited my sentence.

I looked forward never looking at the scale, and as I quickly removed myself after what seemed a lifetime, I quickly put my shoes on and excused myself, never hearing the results. I zigzagged through all my opponents nearly crashing into one of them like I was an ALL-TIME great running back. It wasn't until an hour later when Mia posted everyone's weight on a dry erase board broken down into a clever weekly spreadsheet of sorts. Everyone circled the board as I did, and of course, instead of perusing through everyone's weight I went directly to mine where it was easy to notice that I outweighed everyone by at least 150-pounds or as I read it 345-pounds exactly. I could see all the nurses including the ones that were fine as fuck. They weren't as fine as Mia, but they were certainly serviceable. They had this look on their faces like "damn" as their index finger would scroll against the whiteboard, and seemingly skipped over my name or gently grazed past mine as their eyes remained and their nervous bodies became overwhelmed with empathy. As I lurked into the background taking an instant glare at my weight, my primary focus was on Mia's face as she went through everyone's name asking each one for their goals for next week's weigh in. I wanted to go first just to get the fuck out of there but of course, busting through like a running back would've caused a scene, and that was not going to happen. So, I just stood there in line while everyone gave modest numbers such as "my goal is to lose 2, or 3-pounds." *What the fuck! How could any of my opponents not try to lose more?* I thought. Finally, it was my turn.

"So, what is the goal, Tre?" Mia asked.

My opponents turned in an "about face" as their stares and focus pierced right through me. I exhaled to break the deathly silence of anticipation and snarled my grin.

"Fifteen pounds!"

Mia smirked as gasps fluttered well past my proclamation.

"15-pounds in a week? Are you sure?" Mia said.

Mia smiled not because of my ridiculous proclamation, but I honestly believed she wanted me to hit that weight, so I could save her from her ass-hole of a boyfriend. Was it superficial on her part? Probably, but that's what I believed was the sad reality. She knew deep in her heart that I'd treat her like the queen she was; she just doesn't want any hippo as a fucking lover, and to be honest if the roles (pun) were flipped, I'd be the same way.

That week I went hard on my diet just so I could impress her when I weighed in. I only lost 8-pounds the first week taking a commanding lead. Unfortunately, I spent all my energy that first week, and by the time the final weigh-in occurred three months later, I had gained 4 overall pounds losing to a girl that only lost 3 combined pounds.

I felt pathetic as Mia, and my sister's faces resembled the day after a loved one had passed. Over the top? Maybe, but for sure I felt like I just passed.

# CALLING AUDIBLES

$\mathcal{G}$ROWING UP, WHEN MY homeboys and I played tackle football on the streets (and yes it was the streets). I was always the quarterback, and I must admit I was pretty great at it. If I wasn't such a slacker maybe I could've tried out for QB1; then again, our then high school QB was All-District so the odds of me ever playing would've been improbable anyways. The reason I bring this up is that as a QB you're often forced to call audibles especially if the defense changes its formation before the play.

As for me, when I went out with a friend or family member, for some strange reason doing a pre-emptive audible never crossed my mind until we got to a location. Sure, I chose a location where the odds of a "bump into" were slim to none, but every so often "calling an audible" just before the snap or arriving at my desired location would be necessary.

\*\*\*

Calling audibles was a near weekly occasion for me. After spending a near decade as a Mexican behemoth, calling an audible became frequent. One of my disappointing moments of calling an audible happened not too long ago.

I came home to visit my parents during the summer break after my first year as a teacher. Needless to say, the break was much needed. I had been home for about a week, and considering I spent the last few years at home "at the bottom of the barrel," and now living on my own, I can say with total conviction that I could never go home again. I'm sorry Mom and Pops, you've been great, but I need to expand my wings, but I digress.

After a week passed, I knew my time home was running weary, and besides, I missed my kingdom in Falfurrias, Texas. Yes, the little town nicknamed "Fal," or "Fal-fungus," or as I appropriately nicknamed it the "Fury." With a small population of about 5 to 6,000 people and known for arresting hip-hop mogul Lil Wayne for having weed when crossing the check-point, this small town had become my home.

So, it was my last night, and one of the perks of being large, reclusive, and living at home is getting to know your family. When I received my settlement from my car accident and was able to take out my family to eat more often, that's when we all got to know one another to the point where we oddly became best friends.

\*\*\*

One day we decided to go for dessert at our local *Dairy Queen*, and the reason why I chose this location was that it was a late Wednesday night around 9:30 p.m. and it was next to *Whataburger.* Now, I know for a Valley resident if not all Texans, anyone would choose *Whataburger* over *Dairy Queen* any day of the week. So, as we approached the parking lot, I hear my mom say, "Look the Guerra's are inside." My heart sank. *Fuck!* Now, the Guerra's weren't really friends of my family, but even worse they were parents of an old flame from high school named Cindy.

Everyone thought Cindy and I were a match made from heaven, but because I was a wanted commodity from "back in the days," it was hard to stay faithful to anyone much less Cindy who was a certified dime piece during my high school era. Not to mention our families at the time grew close. As for Cindy, she married after college and had the clichéd life that I'm sure she always wanted: the suburban home, white picket fence, three kids, a dog and a family SUV. As for me, well you've made it this far in the book.

As my pops put the car in park, my mind flooded with ways to get out of there. I sorted through each excuse or scenario resembling Peyton Manning calling an audible while Ray Lewis and the ball-hawking Ravens defense shifted into a sweet poetic flow of fury and elusiveness. The way I shuffled through ways to get out of this potential disaster resembled the great Peyton Manning, except instead of calling "OMAHA! OMAHA!" I partitioned through ideas like Tom Cruise in *Minority Report* and called a play.

"Oh, shit ma!" I said.

"Yes, mijo," Mom said.

"Let me take this call." I pointed to my phone in duress.

"I'll be right in. Here is my debit card. Get whatever you guys want." I said as I shuffled through my wallet paranoid.

I was grateful for technology or else this would've never happened, and I would have been forced to blurt out another location and say something to the effect of "I don't want ice-cream anymore," or something else that my parents would never buy. But because my mom had just mentioned Cindy's parents, the cat would've been out of the bag because they would've known that I was simply lying and didn't want to be embarrassed.

My parents walked into the *Dairy Queen*, and instead of ordering they would let people pass through waiting for me as I faked this phone call. *Shit!* echoed through my mind. *What do I do?* To give my parents the illusion that I might take a while and that they should go ahead with their order, I literally laid back in the car seat for the next half hour and mimed a phone call which felt like an eternity.

Beads of sweat immediately presented themselves as I stayed baking in a routinely hot R.G.V. night just so I could avoid a "bump into" from Cindy's parents, and avoid what would certainly be the greatest version of "spectacle eyes" since my bump into with Lauren. It wouldn't be hard to imagine what their thoughts would've been such as: "Wow! That's a big boy" or "Thank God Cindy didn't marry him." Or "That's what he gets for leaving Cindy." A small part of me always felt that the way I hurt Cindy was why I'm huge in the first place– karma is a motherfucker.

Another 20 minutes passed. "What the fuck!" I shouted in my car appearing as if I was getting pissed at whomever I was foolishly trying to pass off in conversation, but in reality, it was because my parents who were normally "eat and run" people; now out of all days decided to eat at their leisure as I sat in their car perspiring, resembling someone who had been doing engine work all day. Also, *Why the fuck hadn't Cindy's parents left? Was God playing a trick on me?* I looked through the window and noticed that both families were sitting so far apart from one another that they probably didn't even cross paths. This was the part where it was better not to poke the bear, and in this case, not risk having that encounter.

My parents finally walked out even before Cindy's parents. I had a choice to make.

1.) Hang-up the phone and apologize or

2.) Bull-shit the conversation the entire way home and pretend I'm on a phone call.

Instead, I would call an audible from the parking lot off Main Street and decide to b.s. a conversation the rest of the way home. To say I wasn't embarrassed to mime a phone call would be a complete lie. Looking back, I'm sure my parents knew of my bullshit, I just hoped they understood. As for audibles, not all audibles work out.

# NICK NACK PATTY WACKS

*W*HEN A PERSON IS transitioning from regular size clothes to plus-size, they begin to understand how precious the little things are that regular sized people take for granted. An example is: not being able to fit into passenger car seats without having to push the seat all the way back. Which then you have to have the back of the chair completely perpendicular or else you're forced to be all belly and have to slide out the door once you're parked. Another example is restaurant booths. As I expressed in a previous chapter, restaurant booths were something I loved back in the days when I would sit against the wall and have my legs extended shooting the shit with my homeboys.

When you hit a certain size, you must become a genius in visual measurements. Such an example is measuring sitting in a booth and praying that there are no drinks on the table, or risk crashing into the booth causing drinks to spill, or even worse, squeezing in and become pinched for the entire dinner. My final example is something that everyone endures probably once a day, and that is dropping literally anything and bending over and trying to pick "IT" up. What is "IT?" Let me explain.

One of the first things to go when you balloon up in size is your flexibility. Now, don't get me wrong, I've seen fellow big dudes and dudettes dance and kick their legs over their head without a single problem, and

I hold those people in deep regard and give nothing but props. But for the majority of us, or specifically me, I went from a guy who was 5'10, 5'11 with the ability to dunk a basketball (only happened twice in my life) to literally dropping a quarter on the floor and saying "fuck-it," and leaving it behind so I didn't run the risk of my back blowing-out, or even worse bending over and displaying my ass-crack the size of our beloved Milky Way. Believe me, it was all too real, and yes, whether it is a quarter, a pen, or some kind of object, an "audible" was called just so I could have the option to pick it up or not.

For instance, if I dropped a sheet of paper while I was in class, I'd either ask some dude to pick it up for me or wait for class to be over, where I'd be the last person in the room, and reach down with all my magnificent glorious butt crack and pick up the damn sheet of paper. Now there are many more examples I could give, but the purpose of this chapter is to express the little things that are taken away once you become a spectacle.

***

I had just transferred to the local University from our smaller community college in McAllen, Texas. I was about three weeks in and getting used to all the walking and routes to get to class. Now, one would assume I would've lost weight from walking throughout my large University, except during my day of school, I'd usually have a barrage of energy drinks and tacos in-between classes adding to my ever-expanding waistline despite the endless walking.

One day before class, I was running short on funds and decided to get a *Snickers* bar from the vending machine. Instead of my usual three-large breakfast tacos (two chorizos and egg, and one huevo ranchero), I had to settle for a sweet breakfast, and A3 was the *Snickers* bar for 75 cents. I stretched my dollar bill so the machine wouldn't spit it out. I placed the dollar into the slot, and it accepted it the first time. *Sweet!* The machine would make this loud click-clack sound making change. I pushed (A3). The change would rattle through the machine, and as the *Snickers* bar spun open to take its magnificent dive. The quarter from my change would bolt out of the dispenser onto the stone pebbled tile. "Fuck me!" I whispered aloud. I grabbed the *Snickers* bar, and in deep contemplation, I decided if I should leave the quarter or put down my bag to assume the position to bend over. Over the top? Nope! This was my reality and my punishment. I mean I would much rather have had a "bump into" with Lauren, Ana or Cindy then pick up that fucking quarter. I called an "audible," and checked if the coast was clear. It is in this moment I realized that I needed to stop being a lazy pussy and pick up that fucking quarter– it was everything to me that I pick it up. I put down my heavy ass bag, stretched and placed my feet in a 90-degree angle from each other, so I could obtain balance to bend over comfortably without running the risk of ripping my shorts, or even worse tumbling over and not being able to get up. I took a deep breath and bent over. With my ass resembling a traffic cone because of my new highlighter orange gym shorts, the groove of my fingertip barely grasped onto the quarter. I swear, if it was a dime I would've been fucked. I flicked the quarter towards me and pivoted to a more comfortable stance to grab the damn coin. I stood straight and jacked up my shorts pulling out the wedge that had enough clearance for a traffic jam to make through. I inhaled like a bodybuilder just squatted 500-pounds and took a bite out of my *Snickers* that I deserved. After I wiped the beads of sweat and smiled with great relief, I turned around, and what appeared to be a petite vision with golden hair and a string of a white pearl smile stood right behind me astonished. My smile instantly swelled to depletion like a broke man paying bills. I stumbled to grab my bag and rushed right past her and tried to avoid eye contact as I realized in that 5-second process that I had perspired enough to drench my shirt.

I walked to class five minutes before it started, and while I was the only one sitting there beating myself up imagining what that dime-piece saw, butt crack and all, I just wanted to call it a day- of course, I would curse her out in my mind thinking *if I was in shape we would've skipped class together and made love to one another well into the afternoon, and never see each other again.* I decided to squeeze out of my desk and skip class to go home. But first.

> *"Hi ma'am, may I order your carne guisada flour tacos?"*
> *"Okay, that's three-large carne guisada tacos. Is that all?*
> *The drive-thru lady asked."*
> *"Can you also throw in a large soda, and two tamales de*
> *pollo?" I asked.*
> *"No problem, will that be all?"*
> *"That will be it, thank you," I said.*

# GOING SOLO

*As* I approached a near decade of physical expansion, I'd become comfortable with doing everything with the company of myself only. During the past two years living in Falfurrias Texas, a mere 60 miles from the chaotic McAllen, Texas I'd been able to remove myself from any possible "bump intos" or "spectacle eyes" because everyone here had always seen me as a rather large man. So, being 60 miles removed I've found my kingdom, and to be honest I loved it.

As I've mentioned in previous chapters, I'd grown accustomed to doing things on my own terms. An example being: eating out alone. Now, normally I'd have my podcasts to listen to. Whether it be *"The Herd"* for my daily sports fix, or *WTF w/Marc Maron*. I would sadly sit alone and envision how great it would be to be at a restaurant on a date or with a buddy while listening to Colin Cowherd speak continuously about LeBron James, or Marc Maron talk about his cats (Boomer lives!) I knew it was pathetic, but I grew accustomed to my own skin and would prefer eating or hanging out on my own.

When I moved to Falfurrias, I made some great friends/teaching buddies, and although they fell in the much-needed void countering my solace, I always preferred to be alone leading me to ask myself: *Is the need for preferring to be alone a residual to being a large man? Or, have I grown so dense to never desire companionship?* To get to my goal of a 180-pounds from my current 317 seemed like such a global conquest that maybe subconsciously, I can't see myself ever wearing a sensible size that I can't help but default to prefer doing everything on the solo, whether it be: going out to eat, going to the movies, or even on trips on my own. My fear of ever being caught while being fat is and will always be my safe space. I can only pray it is not.

# IV
..
# DEATH
*of a junky*

# AIN'T NO WAY

*J*UNE 1, 2012 SHOULD be labeled "the worst day of my life." What makes this specific day unique to me was the moment of euphoria I experienced after getting t-boned by a drunk driver. Whenever I tell my story of when I got t-boned, I'm always asked. "How did I survive?" and that's when I realize that there is no way I could label this near tragedy as "the worst day of my life."

May 31, 2012 was like any other day, except the first of the month was looming, so naturally, it felt like a perfect time to begin a diet... again. During this period of my life, I had just crossed the 350-pound barrier and knew I had to do something. After spending this Thursday afternoon watching motivational videos on *YouTube*, I suddenly had the urge to attack this diet full-force. There was something about this day that I honestly felt that the next day I was going to challenge myself and conquer this diet and get back to my old weight.

June 1st was here. I waited until 4 a.m. to go to my local *Wal-Mart* Superstore to shop for supplies so I could begin my diet. I decided to do the low-carb diet because that is what worked for me the first time from when I weighed 282-pounds.

Before I left for *Wal-Mart*, I tip-toed out of my house like the (sumo) ninja I am. I checked to see if my parents light under their door was on, and silently walked out the door for what should've been my last time.

While shopping, I bought mounds of steak fajita, chicken breast, *San Manuel* chorizo, cans of tuna, *Spam*, and of course eggs amongst other low-carb foods. While walking the aisles of infinite food possibilities, I came across the frozen food section and saw *DiGiorno's* Pizza calling my name. The thought of *this would be the perfect food to end my half-decade of excessive consumption because the 1st of the month was here, and because of those silly motivational YouTube videos, I knew that I was primed for a phoenix-like ascension towards "Skinnyville."* I grabbed the *DiGiorno's* pizza and checked out as quickly as possible ready to tackle June 1st with full authority.

After I put the bags of food behind the front seat of my car, I attached the auxiliary cord to my phone, so I could listen to some motivational music on the way home. Now, *Wal-Mart* is about a 5-minute drive from my parents' home, so I decided to put on my favorite Aretha Franklin song which is "Ain't No Way"—it was perfect for the ride.

The roads were empty. All that kept me company was the sleepy houses, and the blinking stars as if they were spying on me personally. Considering I was the only one cruising the streets as Aretha and Cissy Houston operatic voices cascaded a sweet hymn to my senses. I became flushed with goosebumps as I whispered along motivated.

I was approaching a red light from a distance and prematurely slowed down. About a hundred feet from the intersection the light turned green. As Cissy Houston's voice hit an octave as high as the stars that were spying on me, I crossed the intersection freely. In an instant, Franklin's voice became mute as a pulverizing roaring crunch of metal crashed upon my senses. Strangely, in that instant, I didn't realize I was in an accident until I comprehended that my car was spinning out of control. As I spun like a top, I shouted in fear to the sky not knowing what was happening. Although this chaos took seconds, it felt like I was spinning for an eternity as I was able to tell myself *"whatever I do, don't hit your head."* I gripped the stirring wheel desperately holding my body in place resisting against the inertia in fear that I don't crush my skull and risk a coma or even worse, death. How shitty would it be to die of a car accident, when I'm out this early in the morning trying to save myself nutritionally?

While screaming to my God and spinning in what had to be four 360s. I was fastly approaching a telephone pole. Of course, my feet were slammed on the breaks, as if it mattered—I embraced for impact. Thankfully, because I was doing everything I could to not hit my head before I slammed onto the pole, I turned my body somewhat to the side as if I was sliding into second base. The front end of my car would resemble the old A-frame from the *Whataburger* fast food joints from back in the days.

As I tried to collect myself and come around to the fact that I was in an accident; sounds of hot fluics dripping onto the dark asphalt overwhelmed my hearing adding to the euphoric fear I was now suddenly enduring. I surveyed my surroundings, and the passenger side was concaved and about a foot away from claiming my end. It suddenly hit me that I had to get out. I tried to open my door, but it was crushed. Frustrated, I sat confused, because the guy who t-boned me hit my car from the passenger side. I pushed my shoulder into the door and couldn't get it open. Suddenly, I heard footsteps patter as I realized that my window had been shattered as some young guy in his early 20s rushed up to my window and asked,

"Are you okay?"

"Yes, just get me out!" I said hysterically.

The guy tries to open my door but can't. I looked up to see who this guy was and his face was red, red with blood as his nose was crushed, and his lip hanging free. This had to be the guy who hit me. I wanted to leap out of my window not only to beat the fuck out of this guy but because I felt like the car was about to explode; which I'm sure is because I had watched too many movies. I tried to lift myself through the window, but I was too heavy to ever get myself out. The guy who hit me ran back to his car, as four other young kids ran to my car witnessing the entire thing.

"Hey man, that guy ran a red and hit you. I can't believe you survived that. WHAT THE FUCK!"

Knowing that I was not at fault somehow calmed me down. As the adrenaline wore off suddenly, I couldn't feel my legs, and my stomach felt like it was on fire. *Oh shit! Please God, don't let me be paralyzed.* I recalled an old friend of mine who died at the age of 12 because he got paralyzed from an accident.

While in a desperate panic as my legs went numb one of the guys asked:

"Hey man, you need me to call someone for you?"

I searched for my phone, and thankfully it remained in the cup holder in the armrest that was now perpendicular to my waist. I quickly check to see if it was working and it was fine. I hand him the phone and tell him to search for "Pops" on my recent calls. As he called, I closed my eyes in fear and frustration because I couldn't feel my legs, and I couldn't get out of this fucking car. A loud fluttering horn pierced through. I opened my eyes to firemen rushing to me with no ambulance in sight. I then remembered that the fire department was less than three blocks away which I couldn't have been more grateful for.

"Sir are you okay?" The fireman asked.

"Um…Yes! But I can't feel my legs." I said.

"Okay, just sit still please, and don't move."

Two firemen desperately tried to open my door but couldn't. Then one of the firemen opens the back-passenger door sliding behind my seat surely stepping on my low-carb meals. *I hope he didn't crush my DiGiorno's pizza.* I thought. The fireman puts his hands on my ears and holds my head in place.

"Please, Sir don't move."

Finally, the ambulance arrived. One of the medics replaced the fireman from my backseat and repeated.

"Please Sir, don't move."

Upon being held still, I took a few breaths to try to calm down when I hear:

"Tre! Tre!"

I open my eyes, and it was Superman.

"Dad!"

"It's going to be okay Sonny!"

Streams of tears rolled down my cheeks as the medic held my head in place. Something about hearing the name Sonny overwhelmed me as it was an endearing nickname my parents called me. The firemen would come rushing to my car with the jaws of life to try and pry open my door that was pinched shut. Even though the sound of the jaws of life overwhelmed any chaos going outside my car, I knew I was safe because Superman was there to calm me.

About 30 minutes would pass until the firemen were able to cut open my door. Thankfully my legs would regain feeling in that time. The ambulance would gently put me on the gurney, put my neck in a brace, and take me to the ambulance. Naturally, my thoughts were, *Do they have the manpower to lift me up?* And in an instant, my question was answered as the fireman had to come to their aid and assist them in taking me into the truck. Before they'd close the door to the ambulance, Superman would tell me "We'll follow you to the hospital, Sonny!" Mom with a whimper in her voice would also shout through "It's going to be okay mijo."

***

The ride to the hospital was surreal in itself. The ambulance had both the other guy and me together in one ride. I thought it was strange as him and I would talk about the San Antonio Spurs blowing a lead to the Oklahoma City Thunder in the Western Conference Finals. Besides apologizing to me profusely as the medic took our blood. I would learn that he hated my Spurs and that his squad was indeed the Thunder which made me hate him even more.

We finally arrived at the hospital, and as they placed me onto the rolling doctor's bed, they parked me aside from the hallway as I assumed the nurse and medic awaited which room to place me in, as it seemed the hospital overflowed with patients. While waiting, Superman appears.

"Are you okay Sonny?" Superman asked.

"I'm so sorry about everything dad."

"I'm just happy you're okay."

Superman hugs me instantly calming me from my near fatal night. As my dad pulled away, I noticed blood on his arm which for an instant I wasn't sure where it was from. I then realized *Holy shit! Am I cut?* I raised my arm thankful that I even had that capability and sure enough my entire arm was soaked in burgundy blood. I took a deep breath of relief as I checked my body for any other bloody wounds—I was clear. Dad would tell me that my brother and mom were waiting for me in the waiting room, while my sister was on her way, which another sense of reassurance came over me as I was grateful for the family support and concern.

While trying to explain to Dad what happened, the medic interrupts our conversation.

"Sir, how much do you weigh?"

Until this moment I had never told anyone how much I weighed. Sure, that day in swimming class was an embarrassing moment for me, but they were perfect strangers. Now, I was about to tell my weight, and because my dad was there awaiting my response, I was now concerned he would look at his once proud son to reveal out loud what I'm sure he already knew, but probably never wanted to hear. After all, just looking at me you'd know I was an obese motherfucker. Now, I had weighed myself earlier that day because I was going to go into the first of the month with a diet plan and wanted to write down my starting weight, so I could measure my weekly progressions. That morning about 20 hours earlier I had weighed 350-pounds. I looked at the medic, and once to Dad, and back again to the medic and said... "about 330-pounds sir." I closed my eyes embarrassed praying that Superman's super hearing went deaf for that second, but I knew he heard everything. I laid there ashamed of my reveal considering that I lied to the doctor about my weight; wishing I never survived that wreck.

"I'm grateful you're okay Sonny, I know mom and your brother are worried sick." Dad said rescuing me from my embarrassing reveal and thankfully changing the subject.

My eyes weld again with tears except this time I tried my best to hold them back.

"Thanks, dad, I'll be honest, I'm happy to be okay too. Also, I'm happy that I didn't shit my pants."

Both Dad and I laughed hysterically as the nurse finally pushed my doctor's bed to my designated room. Before we entered the room, the medic would stop and discuss my accident with another nurse as he grabbed my file. Both Dad and I waited in silence when the nurse asked the medic pushing my cart.

"He's coming from a bad car accident?" While whispering.

"Yeah, he's lucky to have survived. His weight probably saved him."

I could tell I wasn't supposed to hear that, as I looked away in shame.

While waiting for the doctor to arrive, my entire family would keep me company crying as I told my version of what happened and how I tried to avoid hitting my head. We'd also laugh talking about old memories. Mom would of course, sit in silence probably shocked to see her big son suddenly vulnerable as she would clean the blood off my arms, neck, and legs. When the doctor arrived three hours later the first thing he stated was.

"Just so you know the man who hit you is on the next floor up. After he is excused to leave he will be taken to jail for drunk driving, and apparently running a red light, texting, and speeding."

Sighs overwhelmed the room, as my mom, and sister began to cry again.

"Honestly, I'm not sure how you survived or at the very least are not paralyzed. If I could guess, I'm sure your weight provided the cushion necessary to absorb such a blow."

I avoided eye contact with my family as he mentioned my weight.

"Let me ask you, did you have your seatbelt on?"

"Yes, of course."

"Well, I'm sure that had a lot to do with it."

The doctor approached me to check my vitals. Then suddenly, in front of my entire family, he did something I wished he'd done in private but instead chose that exact moment when I was still emotional from his diagnosis of how I survived and pulled up my shirt in front of my family without warning.

Until this exact moment, I believe the last time my family ever saw me without a shirt was the first time they brought me home the day after my birthday 31 years earlier. Of course, as he lifted my shirt, I looked up and away because the last thing I wanted to see was the expression of their son's blubbery bulbous body as he lifted my shirt to my chin like he was revealing the Elephant Man, and everything hanging in all of its magnificent glory.

"I see that the seat belt left a mark on your entire chest and indented your stomach."

I nod while looking away. My family on the other hand never gasped in astonishment or whispered words in response to what they just saw. As far as I could tell with my eyes pinched shut, I'm sure they quickly grinned, and out of respect to me acted as if they were normal. The doctor would go on about how my weight and seatbelt probably saved my life while my shirt remained raised, and my rotund bruised body remained exposed.

I would go home later that morning stiff as a board and dose myself with meds. After the painkillers kicked in, I was able to slowly walk to the restroom mirror and check out the damage, and for the first time in years, I wanted to see my reflection. Since my back was stiff and I was hunched over, it was painful to take off my shirt. With the pain being too overwhelming even with painkillers, I would hang my shirt off my neck, and straighten my back as much as possible to see what the cocksucka did to me. The seatbelt had left a perfectly purple bruising across my entire body causing an actual seatbelt shape indention across my gut which until this day is still there. It's as if, my gut was sectioned in half.

I would go through months of physical therapy as I had apparently damaged my back permanently. According to the doctor, when I resisted my body from hitting my head, the force of the car accident and my resistance caused my back to twist unnaturally, and most likely lead me to a lifetime of back issues, and surely ending my basketball career—which to be honest had been on the back burner anyway.

I later learned that the drunk driver who hit me was driving 60 miles per hour, and texting. Even though he would serve that weekend in jail, he'd endure a broken nose, and a stitched-up lip, without having insurance. When we'd go to the courthouse, the Judge would rule in favor of him, because he was also a Navy shipman. The Judge would require that he return to San Diego and complete his Naval training hoping he'd grow up and become a responsible man. The Judge would then turn to me and state:

"Son, I'm sorry for your accident, be thankful that you were insured and please use that money for any future treatment you may need. You're both dismissed."

I limped out of the courtroom, as the man who hit me nonchalantly walked out never recognizing me. Although I was hoping for some kind of acknowledgment from the Judge, and somehow make the dude who hit me pay some kind of consequence, I realized that I should be blessed to be alive.

I did collect some money from my insurance in future months. In this time, I couldn't work and was forced to take online classes as it was a pain in the ass just to get out of bed. As much as I'd love to say I spent that year eating better because of my life lesson in that car accident, that wasn't the case. If I'm not mistaken, I had breached 375-pounds by years end and was officially a lost cause.

Looking back, I've always felt that this accident was God's way of telling me to get started and start your life again. Unfortunately, that never came. If anything, I would use this accident for years as an excuse as to how I lost my way when in reality I had been lost for a long time.

I'm not sure if I should be grateful that my weight was the reason why I survived this crash, but I know for damn sure there ain't no way I could survive long being this weight.

# SOMETIMES, IT'S HOW HARD YOU FALL

*L*IFE AS A STATISTICAL spectacle has its humbling experiences. For me, I've had numerous as I have written in previous chapters. Also, to go along with humbling experiences are those unexpected moments where life not only hits you as hard as Tyson in his zenith; that it forces you as a person to take in account your life that led to this exact moment, but also makes you want to change your life or not.

I was about six years into my obesity when "IT" happened. Now, I've had variations of this happening, and "IT" had never been a problem until this day.

It was an unassuming day. I arrived home from picking up some grub, granted it was during the daytime on a random Tuesday or Wednesday so the odds of a "bump into" were slim to none— besides I was going through the drive-thru so when I came home with two or three bags of saturation my entire family would be at work, so I didn't have to worry about any "spectacle eyes" from my family.

I pulled up to my driveway and saw my little brother Jesse who is ten years younger than me working out in the garage with the garage door halfway open.

*Fuck!* I shouted in the car while unplugging my auxiliary cord from my phone. It was time to call an audible. Now, my little brother Jesse also had trouble with weight, and thankfully had never come anywhere close to my size. Because of his short stature, he had to work hard just to keep a decent weight. Now, by no means was I ever a great brother to him growing up, and I have repeatedly apologized to him for leaving him stranded during his adolescence. Jesse has forgiven me, but I've always felt incompetent in nature when it comes to making up for my immaturity during his maturation.

I sat in the car for a split second *"Rolodexing"* through my ideas of how to get away with walking into the house with these many bags of food. I called my audible, and although the garage was halfway up covering my brother's upper torso, there would be no way he would see me with bags of food. Also, by the way his feet were moving to the beat of his *P90X*, I could possibly get away by sneaking in like the ninja that I am. I decided to call another audible, and grab my bags, and make a break for it. One step out of my car, and I was keeping an eye on Jesse hoping he didn't break stride, so I could indulge myself in bliss in my bedroom. I clutched onto both bags, and Jesse was still going toe to toe with Horton. I reached into my car to grab my soda, and because of my lack of flexibility, I was forced to take my eyes off Jesse. I quickly grabbed the soda, and upon looking back at the garage, my brother's feet seemed to have disappeared. *Fuck!* I shouted in my head. I call a third audible truly reflecting Peyton Manning except instead of shouting "Omaha! Omaha! Omaha!" I'm shouting in my head *Fuck! Fuck! Fuck!* I didn't have time to shuffle through my mental *Rolodex* of excuses, so upon seeing a blitz formation from Ray Lewis and perennial defensive end Terrell Suggs (should've won the Heisman), I noticed the proverbial play clock dwindling down 3,2,1... I make a decision based on reflex. I decided to put the bags down in the driver's seat and my soda back figuring I'll just come back for them. *Fuck!* I closed my door and decided to go into the garage and check for damage control leaving my food behind risking it getting cold. The garage door was lower than expected, so I rolled under, and that's when "IT" happened.

I was on the other side of the garage, and I'd see Jesse near the DVD player changing discs. After I rolled under the garage, "IT" hit me like a ton of bricks. I couldn't stand up. It was as if the entire mass of the Earth was attached to my waist. I looked at my brother who was completely focused on his DVDs; luckily, he didn't notice I was literally the human version of a beached whale behind him. I tried to play it off as I just sat there paralyzed.

"What up dawg? How many sessions have you done?" I asked hoping he didn't notice his once "badass" brother was now a lost cause struggling to simply stand. Jesse just nodded and continued his workout focused. Thankfully, it was cold outside, so I wasn't sweating struggling to find a way to stand up, but I knew my food would be getting cold, and my fries would be on the verge of turning to shit, so I had to figure something out, and soon. I searched around to find something to help assist me, and I was on an island. I couldn't believe there was nothing there to help me get on my feet. *How was I going to pull myself up?* I thought. My core felt like sandbags, and my arms and legs had since resembled a beige cool-whip dimpled casserole.

Jesse was in full swing never acknowledging me. *Jesus, I wish I had his focus.* But I needed to focus. I took a second to strategize, and instead of calling another audible, I just sat there stumped. I knew I had over thought everything as I was kicking myself for hesitating in the first place, and not making a run for it when I had a chance. To say that this audible was a humbling experience— of course it was, especially since I was discovering something new about myself for the first time that I didn't know was even possible, and it was physical.

I had to decide to either roll over to a chair about three full body rolls from me or do a butt slide— which I'm sure would've resembled a dog sliding his butt across the carpet just to wipe-ass; except for me, it would be just so I could stand the fuck-up. I decided to slide over, one slide and I was done. My gelatinous arms from the slide over had given out, and now I didn't have the strength to push myself up from the garage floor—I was fucked. My only option was to roll over, but I didn't want to be seen by my little brother. Imagine those "spectacle eyes." He would lose all respect for me if he hadn't already. Suddenly, it hit me. I shouted out to Jesse.

"Dude, can you help me up? I rolled my ankle." Doing this and referring to my old basketball injury from my "heyday," had been a running joke in my family that I would often use to get out of a chore or an assignment. Jesse rushed to me while never breaking stride in his workout. I extended my hand, bracing my body to assist in a full-body yank from Jess to somehow not appear to weigh as much as I did. In one quick swoop Jesse pulled me up, and I was free, and Jesse went back to his workout never expressing or saying anything. Did he know I was bullshitting and unable to get up? Who knows? All I knew was that it was time to get my grub on and pray my fries weren't cold.

> *"Yes! May **WE** order your triple deluxe cheeseburger combo?*
> *I asked.*
> *"No problem, is there anything else you'd like to add to your*
> *order?" The drive-thru attendant asked.*
> *"Um…can you also add your 2 for 1 hot dogs with extra*
> *packets of mustard?"*
> *"Okay, anything else?" The drive-thru attendant asked.*
> *"Yes, can you add a large banana-split dessert?"*
> *"No problem."*

# VANISHING ACT

$\mathcal{P}$ARTS OF THIS BOOK may seem like an apology tour. You must understand, life as a large man you either become submissive and take the hits from those with "spectacle eyes" or being called a "fat fuck" for the sake of not being a recluse— which I give major props for those having the bravery for being free while being exposed for which I could never attain. Another aspect would be turning into a reclusive depressed person where you become so isolated that you burn bridges with friends or family knowing damn well they would never judge you in the first place, but because of outside forces and insane insecurities you would much rather stay in, call an "audible" and call it a day.

I can honestly say that we would much rather prefer the latter and be of a decent size just so we could laugh and love with everyone without worrying if a "bump into" was about to occur, or even worst skip-out on a family or friends event risking everything all for the sake of "isola- tional-bliss," and self-indulge all while your loved ones wonder "Where the fuck is Tre?"

I understand that there are worst things in life and that many people would love to switch places with me, but for me during this period of my life (and still currently) life got tough. The school year was ending which meant one thing. A "murderer's row" of birthdays and anniversaries were coming up. I swear it's like my family planned this shit out knowing one day I'd become a fat-fuck and be forced to eat birthday cakes, and attend dinner parties making it impossible to diet, and worst of all the fucking non-stop pictures. I knew my parents and family had the best intentions, but they had to know that any fat fuck would dread the idea of being in front of a camera. So, of course, an "audible" would ensue, and I do my best to clamor to the back of photos so the bodies in front would cover me, and somehow camouflage the obese motherfucker in the background as much as possible. And to add a cherry on top with the invention of social media, I knew my family would post those pics for everyone to see like that DREADFUL day of my college graduation a year later a.k.a. "Worst Day of My Life." Imagine, those family friends poking the "like" button or choosing the "agape smiley face" because of the walrus standing in the background behind my family like I was really fooling anyone. Paranoid? Maybe, narcissistic? Without a doubt, but a fat fuck had to survive somehow no matter how petty.

With the onslaught of family events to come, it was time for my amazing niece's first birthday. By now, I'd experienced my parents' anniversary, Mother's Day, Mom's birthday, all before my niece's birthday in early July, so it was safe to say I'd gained more weight and had taken endless photos.

My "audible" for the summer was to take summer classes, so I could have a way to duck out of the summer events and have an excuse to not be present in any more family parties. The problem was all these events just so happened to take place during the weekend including my niece's birthday party. So, my family decided to have a family-only dinner at my sister's home during the week and then the friends and extended family edition on the weekend. *Great!* I thought. My thinking was, I'd go to the family event and then break the "bull-shit" news that I have some school commitment that I couldn't get out of for the weekend party.

Do I know I should be there? Of course, but the then current "demon" completely absolved any empathetic feeling I may have had at the time, and to be honest still currently have.

For this occasion, I knew I was fucking-up. I mean for Christ's sake it was my baby niece's 1st birthday. Will she remember I wasn't there? No, but my family would for damn sure, but in my mind, I'd much rather get chewed out by my sister and family then see a relative I hadn't seen in ages or even worse see my sister's co-workers ogling me with their "spectacle eyes" and thinking in the realm of "Wow! That's a big boy, no I wouldn't fuck him." Sad but true.

I decided to rent a hotel in the city informing my family I had to leave town for a school assignment letting my sister know that I may make it, but for the tail end of the party. My sister was totally cool with this. Did I ever intend on showing up? Hell-no! If there was any consolation, I did cry about not being there for my niece, but I had zero mental capacity to ever face whatever would've been waiting for me that weekend.

After my tears soaked, I did divulge freely without coming home trying to hide my greasy addiction and enjoyed my night in solitary freedom at the hotel. In retrospect, I know I was selfish, but I knew then that hiding out was my only way of self-peace— I'm sorry

\*\*\*

My relationship with my sister Karina was different from my relationship with my brother Jesse. For a stretch of time, it was only my sister and me, and besides the usual hi-jinx between brother and sister such as our family trip to *Disneyland* when I was 9 years old, my sister and I were close. This is why as a then 32-year old man, I cried and wept after leaving my sister and niece high and dry. I will admit, I fell asleep in my hotel with candy and burger wrappers surrounding me, but when I

ÉÉÉÉÉÉÉ

woke-up the guilt devoured any selfish cell I had remaining in me, and I instantly knew I had to make it right.

I called my sister, and I was immediately met with deserving sighs and contrite one-word responses as I asked her if she could come over, so I could talk to her. Of course, she wasn't feeling it, but as I explained myself without giving it all away, by the kindness of her heart she agreed to come by Mom's house, so I could somehow explain my absence.

In anticipation for my sister arriving for the apology of the century, I'll be honest I wasn't sure what to expect. After a much-needed shower, I must've stared at my reflection endlessly with regret and remorse. I recalled a much older co-worker I once worked with tell me about the first time she saw her reflection in a mirror and didn't recognize herself. Although she felt youthful in mind and spirit, her body had changed. Considering she spent her entire life embracing her vanity, she didn't know what she was looking at despite the fact she had spent the night before embracing her reflection. Devastated, she would come within an inch of the mirror, and discover lines, and stretched skin she had never noticed before. Shocked at what she was looking at, streams of tears would trickle down coating her newly discovered crevices. As minutes turned into hours, she would stare passed her vacant reflection realizing that what she was looking at was inevitable, and never happened overnight, but was always there. I could say the same looking at my reflection for what seemed like the first time in ages. As I've mentioned before when your body resembles a gelatinous pool of "beige saturation" mirrors become obsolete. But this *moment* when I was in a deadlock "stare down" with my toughest competition, I saw what my bad-habits had done to my once youthful face. Besides the obvious double chins and a hot dog pack in the back of my neck, my damaged creased skin overwhelmed me. Instead of my crinkly wrinkled face being mistaken for wisdom, the deep lines told stories of my years as a fast food junky.

As I washed my face hoping for a miracle skin rejuvenation, I heard the door slam knowing my sister was finally here — *SHOWTIME!* I exited the restroom, and my sister was there with my brother-in-law and my little brother. *Jesus fuck! It's going to be a true apology tour.*

I took a seat on my *Lazy Boy* that I was barely able to fit into and greeted everyone.

"Hey guys, thanks for coming," I said.

"What's up, bro? How was your assignment for school? We missed you at Maya's birthday party," my big sister said.

I was caught off guard, I was expecting and strangely hoping for a deserving tongue lashing, but my sister seemed sincerely happy to see me.

"I know, and that's why I want you guys here, please sit," I said nervously.

My sister showed me pictures of my precious little angel Maya's birthday party. Maya's glee during her important milestone was as if wisdom and love were fully embraced on her first birthday celebration. Her eyes and smile emphasized any form of happiness that had ever existed on this Earth, and I missed it, I missed all of it. My neck drooped as I broke into tears publicly for the first time since my dog "Casper the G.O.A.T." passed away New Year's Eve of 2008. Surprisingly, my brother-in-law Jacob rushed to my aid. I was eternally grateful and thankful for his presence.

"What's the matter?" Jacob asked.

I tried talking but with every word I spoke came with patters of air and tears as the image of my niece smiling overwhelmed me.

"I lied," I said in a whimper.

"What do you mean?" My big sister asked.

I opened my eyes wiping away my tears. Now, everyone huddled around me. Jesse, my big sister Karina, and Jacob. I looked into their eyes, and I saw their deepest concern, and it caused me to bury my head back into my palms in complete disappointment. A flash of Maya's infinite smile suddenly became overwhelmed with the concerned eyes of my siblings. *How could I have hurt them?* I said in my head.

"I'm so sorry," I said while sputtering.

"Sorry? You don't have to be sorry." My little brother Jesse said.

I felt the closeness and the bond that I have always craved from my little brother. I took in a deep breath and garnered the strength to talk. I raised my head from the depth of my lap.

"I had no assignment." I looked at my sister's face expecting a look of disappointment, but she never took her eyes off me.

"I'm just so embarrassed about everything; I've become scared to be seen." As I talked, there were no "audibles" being called to save me? I'm not sure if I was speaking from the heart or was on auto-pilot, but everything I said was in its sincerity the truth, and to be honest was soul cleansing. I apologized continuously while also telling them about my self-diagnosis of being depressed.

"I'm so tired of hiding and hurting everyone." I blurted in tears.

Everyone cried with me as I felt the synergy from my siblings. Jacob put his arm around me as both my little brother and older sister latched on to me as if we all knew the only way to help me was to be together, and we were impenetrable. At that *moment,* I had felt the presence of God in the extension of his greatest creation— FAMILY.

We talked the entire night telling old stories of our childhood and laughed the night away. Needless to say, I was forgiven without ever being talked about, and since I decided no matter where I am physically, mentally, or emotionally, I will never miss another family occasion.

We began a diet (my brother, sister, and I) and had fun with it.

Although we wouldn't complete our goals, we not only built bridges for our relationships, but reinforced them, and I'm grateful for what I have with them.

> *"It must be nice to disappear*
> *To have a vanishing act*
> *To always be looking forward*
> *And never looking back*
> *How nice it is to disappear*
> *Float into a mist"* –
> **"Vanishing Act"** by: Lou Reed

# THE BUCKET LIST

*I* WILL ADMIT THAT I never knew what a "bucket list" was until I saw the damn movie when it premiered more than a few years ago. Of course, after watching this film, I had the certain urge to write such a list. Sure, I've written goals before, but since I've seen this movie sadly my bucket list had only consisted of "what and when" as in when I'll lose weight rather than run a marathon, complete a triathlon, do a *Spartan* race, make a hundred free throws in a row (closest I ever got was 91 out of a 100) which occurred the first time I lost that first 100-pounds a near decade earlier. After many variations of this bucket list, I realized that this list was becoming more and more impossible especially after I hit the 350-pound marker and 401-pounds loomed the following year.

After reaching 401-pounds and experiencing the worst day of my life (my graduation,) my bucket list only consisted of one thing: SURVIVE TO 40. With all this insane "yo-ycing" going from my high school weight of a 165-pounds to 282-pounds to 175-pounds, then ballooning up from 175 to 301-pounds, then from 301-pounds to 231-pounds, to 231-pounds to my worst 401-pounds, then from 401 to 313 to 365, and finally as I complete this sentence on July 5, 2018 317-pounds. I wouldn't be surprised if I knocked 25 to 35 plus years of expectancy. Would I love to one day accomplish all those physical feats on my bucket list? Of course, but I need to survive and get back to a 179-pounds and simply live a healthy lifestyle, hopefully recouping the many years I've shredded– if possible.

It's interesting because as a large man you understand the threat of death and realize that you're only a moment away from dying as it is to any regular civilian across the globe. But to know that our addiction can claim us, causes us to ask ourselves "Is this our last meal?" There were situations where I cleaned up my apartment thinking my last breath was looming because of mixing depression with a smorgasbord of fried foods while also not having stepped outside for fresh air in weeks. Imagine the concoction of funk permeating through my apartment.

The bucket list became a document of foresight, but without ever having the insight to fight for what was on my list. As of recent years, the bucket list has morphed into plans I could physically do while I transition to hopefully a medium shirt such as: earn my master's degree in Mexican history and eventually my doctorate. Another reachable aspect I have on my bucket list is getting closer to my brother, going to a Yankee, Spurs, Longhorns, and Cowboy games with my family, and of course, traveling the world. The great thing about this list is that it's all achievable, and I certainly plan on checking off every one of those boxes especially the family goals all while reaching my physical pursuits as well, and most importantly recouping my lost years– if possible.

# CLIMBING EVEREST...TWICE

$\mathcal{B}$Y THE TIME YOU get to this chapter, most readers will probably believe I'm undisciplined or in search of empathy, while others might claim I'm simply trying to survive. Are these self-inflicted wounds? Perhaps, but I believe the better question is "Are those self-inflicted wounds well deserved?"

Another theme throughout this book is my claim that I'm dealing with addiction. Is addiction real? Or an excuse? You often hear the many success stories and failures of alcoholics and drug addicts, and I honestly feel obesity has its place amongst the tiers of addiction. Whenever I've tried to look for some kind of rehab or A.A. version for obesity, it usually consists of some kind of resort or physical trainer who's never experienced a day of being large. Like I've mentioned throughout this book, my family has been my only support system and I love them deeply for it. I feel blessed to have had them as a resource throughout my addiction, but even I feel embarrassed trying to categorize myself as any kind of addict, because I'm not sure my addiction is even real as silly as that may sound. All I know is that when I'm alone, I have no self-control and at times my appetite will get out of hand, and I can't stop eating. It's scary. There are days where I have great self-control, but in all honesty, I can't reason with my silly cravings as I'm completely consumed with "What am I going to eat?"

Considering I have a college minor in Kinesiology, I have never done any study about obesity, but enduring it for 10 plus years, I can say that I'm an expert when it comes to the pitfalls of being an obese person. This book I'm writing is about the trials and many tribulations I've endured instead of researched-based analysis. Also, this book is for those who don't understand what an obese person thinks or constructs so that the people without this curse can maybe recognize the torture someone like me is going through, instead of having "spectacle eyes" and merely judging. Then again, maybe that's what we need: to be judged, and laughed at so much that we break down and resurrect and put away our crutch and simply begin to move.

By no means does this book have a happy ending. Maybe that will be volume II– if I'm so lucky to publish a second part. As I've hinted in previous chapters, I indeed wrote a majority of these pages at my local *McDonalds* in the small town of Falfurrias, Texas between 10-11:30 p.m. almost every night, and I promise you while writing I was never eating a damn salad.

As I conclude this book, I currently weigh 317-pounds a solid 84-pound lost since I hit my pathetic pinnacle of 401-pounds four years earlier. Yes, it has taken me four years to lose 84-pounds, or as I like to refer to it as my first of two Mount Everest expeditions.

If there is any optimism in this book, it is that I know I'll weigh a 180 pounds recouping some of the years I may have lost because of my current physical status. It's in this climb to the summit that I'll conquer Everest twice, except this time I'll enjoy the view.